Caring for People in Community & Health Services

Frankie O'Sullivan

**with contributions from
Moira Burns and Rachel O'Sullivan**

Gill & Macmillan

D1078698

Gill & Macmillan
Hume Avenue
Park West
Dublin 12
with associated companies throughout the world
www.gillmacmillan.ie

978 07171 5627 6

Print origination by Síofra Murphy
Printed by GraphyCems, Spain
Index by Adam Pozner

The paper used in this book comes from the wood pulp of managed forests. For every tree felled, at least one tree is planted, thereby renewing natural resources.

A CIP catalogue record is available for this book from the British Library

This book is dedicated to Neil, a 16-year-old man with cerebral palsy who changed the direction of my career and my life. – *Frankie O'Sullivan*

With love to John, Paul, Mark, Sean, Damien, Brendan and Catherine. To my daughters-in-law Majella, Yasmeen and Emma and to my grandchildren Ashling, Conor, Kieran and Declan. – *Moira Burns*

Acknowledgements

I wish to express heartfelt thanks to all those who worked with me to produce this book. Thanks to my husband, John, and children, Lauren, Samuel and Roisin, for your patience and support. Thanks to Linda Finegan for all your help with this book and support in 2012. Thanks to Moira Burns and Rachel O'Sullivan for agreeing to write and for making it a painless experience. Thanks to Una O'Hare at Irish Times Training for all her support in 2012. Thanks to Marion O'Brien, Catherine Gough, Kristin Jensen and all the staff at Gill & Macmillian. Finally, thanks to my parents for a lifetime of support and encouragement. – *Frankie O'Sullivan*

First and foremost I would like to thank my husband, John, for his constant love, encouragement and support for my new ventures. I know how they can disrupt life. The same also applies to our children, Paul, Mark, Sean, Damien, Brendan and Catherine. I would like to thank Frankie O'Sullivan for asking me to collaborate with her on this book – it has been a pleasure working with her. Finally, I would like to thank the numerous students I have had the privilege of teaching over the last 20 years – I have learned a lot from them and this has helped with my writing. I hope I have inspired them in their education and that this book will continue to inspire future students in their education as social care practitioners. – *Moira Burns*

Thank you to the following individuals, without whose contributions and support my chapter would not have been written. Frankie, thank you for giving me the opportunity to contribute to the book and supporting me throughout the process. To my parents, Mary and Jerome, and my partner, Niall, thank you for your support and reassurance. – *Rachel O'Sullivan*

Contents

Overview xi

Chapter 1 Care Provision and Practice 1
Moira Burns

Chapter 2 Understanding Ageing 29
Frankie O'Sullivan

Chapter 3 Disability Awareness 53
Rachel O'Sullivan

Chapter 4 Equality and Disability 85
Frankie O'Sullivan

Chapter 5 Understanding Mental Health 99
Frankie O'Sullivan

Chapter 6 Therapeutic Communications:
Knowledge for CCAs 117
Frankie O'Sullivan

Chapter 7 Work Experience 135
Moira Burns

Overview

This text brings into focus three domains of care that are essential to all community care assistants (CCAs) working with vulnerable people in Irish society. Increasingly, more and more people are being cared for within the community in Ireland. This trend is set to continue as the demand for care services increases into the 21st century. In years to come, the demand for community care assistants who can provide care for three particular groups of people – older people, people with disabilities and people with mental health difficulties – will increase. As the social model prevails, more and more people will be cared for in the community.

With the professionalisation of social care, there is a need for clarity across multidisciplinary teams. CCAs are expected to work within the multidisciplinary team and need to be confident and competent in their care practice. In order to deliver on those expectations, CCAs also have specific needs, which include training, support and supervision.

Chapter 1 sets out to formalise the process of caring in the community and identifies the models and theories that underpin care practice. The social model of health, the six dimensions of health and holistic care are introduced in this chapter and further integrated throughout the book. Further integration of the learning outcomes for care support is evident in this chapter in particular, but also throughout the entire book.

Chapter 2 will assist in developing your understanding of older people and the challenges faced by people ageing in Ireland today. We will consider the physical, emotional and social processes of ageing. As we age our propensity to develop a mental health problem as well as structural and functional difficulties increases. Some individuals may even develop a disability in later years. Over the next 30 years, the number of people aged over 65 will double. With fewer people dying of infectious diseases, more people will live for longer with chronic illnesses.

Chapter 3 explores a wide range of physical and intellectual disabilities. Chronic illness, hidden disability and traumatic brain injury are among the many topics discussed.

Chapter 4 discusses concepts of stereotyping, prejudice and discrimination and how this impacts on people with disabilities in a care context. It is intended to assist in the exploration of personal prejudices and enhance understanding of direct, indirect, unconscious and institutional inequalities that occur in society and in care contexts.

Chapter 5 introduces the broad topic of caring for people with mental illness in an understandable way and demonstrates that mental health is a continuum experienced by all. It will identify some common conditions and their signs and symptoms as well as strategies for meeting individuals' needs.

Communication is a core skill in care work and it is essential that care courses have a specific focus on communication within a care setting. Communication involves the exchange of information through the spoken and written word and is a fundamental component of care practice and effective interpersonal skills. It is essential that all CCAs understand the importance of documentation and its role in caring for a vulnerable person, and this is discussed in Chapter 6.

As work experience is a mandatory module, we have included it in Chapter 7 to increase understanding of the importance of reflective practice. Mentoring has been emphasised as a vital component of the work experience module in care practice. Our objective is to enhance quality of care through reflection and supervision, weaving together the core elements of this award and integrating care support.

Settings are an important cornerstone for successful health promotion, as outlined in the 1986 Ottawa Charter. All residential settings for older people and people with disabilities must comply with and maintain the HIQA standards as part of their work practice. A common thread throughout this text is the link with these standards, which must be integrated into training to enhance understanding at student level.

This text is intended to support students who are studying for the FETAC 5 full award 5M4467 and 5M4468 Community and Health Services. This award is increasing in popularity in Ireland due to the broad spectrum of modules available. Modules have been chosen for this text following consultation with community and health services in Ireland that require staff with knowledge and understanding of older people, people with disabilities and people with mental health difficulties. The Care of the Person with Mental Illness module must be chosen as a general studies module. This text will also be useful for those who are studying for the FETAC 5 award 5M4339 in Healthcare Support.

For the purposes of this text, the care worker unit is addressed within Chapter 7 on work experience. The title of community care assistant (CCA) will be used in this text. Where health care worker (HCW) is used, it refers to HCWs in general.

We hope you enjoy reading this text and find it to be an informative guide to assist you in your studies. As committed tutors in the health and social care industry, we have endeavoured to make this material readable, easy to understand and informative.

1
Care Provision and Practice

INTRODUCTION

In this chapter, two aspects of care practice are considered: the people who need care and care itself. The purpose of this chapter is to open up the wider aspects of care and encourage students to explore the models of health, theories and processes that underpin care practice.

There will be some overlap with other chapters and it is preferable to read this chapter in conjunction with Chapter 6 (Therapeutic Communications) and Chapter 7 (Work Experience).

KEY TERMS

- community care assistant (CCA)
- dimensions of holistic health
- disability
- ethnicity
- health promotion
- knowledge
- legislation
- medical model of health
- multidisciplinary team (MDT)
- policy
- qualities
- skills
- social model of health
- statutory/voluntary organisation
- World Health Organisation (WHO)

TRENDS IN HEALTH CARE

We all have the capacity to care and most of us care for and about a number of people during our lives. It is a subject that most of us can readily identify with to such an extent that some decide to enter a caring profession. A capacity to care was often a 'good enough' trait on which to base entry to a caring position, which led to care that was often excellent but could also be ad hoc, irregular or abusive. There was very little emphasis on or understanding of the burdens of care that can be placed on CCAs or the repercussions of that burden on individuals and their families. It is now accepted that each CCA needs training, education, supervision and support in care practice so that a high standard of care is delivered to the individual and that CCAs are supported while being accountable for their care practice. It is no longer acceptable to carry out a task because 'she told me to do it' – or worse, not to carry out certain practices because 'nobody told me to do it'. Care must be planned, evaluated and based on evidence of best practice. In this chapter all of the elements involved in this process will be considered. By the end, students will be in a position to deliver high-quality, holistic health care.

Initially, care needs to be contextualised, and although an in-depth exploration of the history and trends relating to care are very interesting and worthy of exploration, we are limited here to a brief summary.

Historically, care was considered women's work and was delivered by women in the community for the community. Knowledge of herbs, the environment and healing was extensive and passed from one generation to the next in the oral tradition. In the 15th and 16th centuries, the significance of science, industry and commerce began to impact on care and this gave rise to the medical model of health, which has remained the strongest model to date. The focus of this model is 'treat and cure', with huge advances being made in diagnostic technology, drug therapies and surgical interventions extending people's life expectancy, quality of life and expectations. This model of health was professionalised and is predominantly delivered through a hierarchical structure of doctors, nurses and ancillary staff.

However, during the 1950s and 60s, people in the disability and feminist sectors began to campaign for a different type of health care – care that acknowledges and accommodates all dimensions of health; that accepts that many disabilities are incurable; that focuses on the individual rather than the condition and ability rather than disability; and that advocates for the removal of societal structures that impede independent living. This became the social model of health. It is embedded in human rights and health promotion and applies to large numbers of people who are being cared for in the community. Depending on the situation, it is delivered through a multidisciplinary team

(MDT) structure consisting of doctors, nurses and health and social care professionals in consultation with, and with the consent of, individuals who need care and their families.

> **Task**
>
> Did you know that until fairly recently, people with disabilities were often not given antibiotics for common infections – on the basis of their disability? Consider the ethics relating to this practice.

Alongside this new model of health came a demand for higher standards, accountability and the regulation of care practice. The professionalisation of social care was formalised in Ireland with the passage of the Health and Social Care Professional's Act in 2005. The implementation of this Act is ongoing and governs the practice of 12 allied health professionals:

+ Clinical biochemist
+ Dietician
+ Medical scientist
+ Occupational therapist
+ Orthoptist
+ Physiotherapist
+ Podiatrist
+ Psychologist
+ Radiographer
+ Social care worker
+ Social worker
+ Speech and language therapist.

Under the Act there is a responsibility to establish a Health and Social Care Council, 12 registration boards and a complaints and disciplinary committee. Professional registers will be maintained and all health and social care education programmes will be approved and monitored.

Within the social model of health, practitioners from both social and medical models work as part of a multidisciplinary team (MDT), so there must be good communication and co-operation between all practitioners.

Community care assistants need to know the roles and responsibilities of the various practitioners and how the team works together. Teams usually work as follows.

+ **Dieticians** assess the individual's nutritional status and draw up a plan to deal with any medical conditions, such as diabetes, high cholesterol or coeliac. They also offer advice and support on obesity, poor appetite and malnutrition as well as advice for people with complications following a stroke, etc.
+ **General practitioners (GPs)** are community-based doctors who care for the general health of their patients. They work closely with the public health nurse in providing front-line care in the community. They will refer the patient to a specialist if necessary.
+ **Health care assistants (HCAs)** work in a number of positions in residential care, community residential homes and hospitals. HCAs usually deliver practical care on a regular, often daily, basis and therefore know the client and their families very well, thus forming an important link in the MDT. CCAs are HCAs who work in the community.
+ **Occupational therapists (OTs)** provide assessments and supports for people to participate as fully as possible in the activities of daily life.
+ **Physiotherapists** assist people who have lost mobility or movement through disability, accident or illness to regain as much independence as possible.
+ **Public health nurses (PHNs)** are employed by the Health Service Executive (HSE), are based in the community and work with a range of clients, including babies, children, older people and people with disabilities. The PHN will provide supervision and support to the community care assistant.
+ **Registered nurses** have trained in general nursing or specialist areas of psychiatry or intellectual disability. General nurses (RGNs), registered nurse intellectual disability (RNID) and registered psychiatric nurses (RPNs) can be based in acute hospitals, day hospitals, training centres or community residential homes for people with mental health difficulties, intellectual disabilities or older people. They provide specialist care and sometimes supervise CCAs in their work.
+ **Social workers** work within community and residential settings with individuals and families who are experiencing social and emotional difficulties. A large proportion of their work within the HSE is with children at risk, fostering and adoptions.

LEGISLATION AND POLICY

Health care is regulated through laws, policies and guidelines. At this stage you don't need to know the details of every law, but you are expected to know that CCAs are governed by health legislation and policy. All health professionals must work within that legislation. A law is different from a policy in that laws **must** be implemented, whereas policies contain the details of how a law **may** be implemented. Laws must go through a strict process and criteria and are difficult and complicated to change, whereas policies can be drawn up and changed fairly easily – for example, in line with changing trends or the advancement of technology.

The following is a list of some of the laws that govern the practice of CCAs in relation to health and groups in society:

- Children's Act 2001
- Mental Health Act 2001
- Equality Act 2004
- Disability Act 2005
- Health and Social Care Professional Act 2005
- Health, Safety and Welfare at Work Act 2005
- Health Act 2007
- Nurses and Midwives Act 2011.

As well as these laws, relevant policies and declarations include:

- UN Declaration of Human Rights, 1948
- UN Declaration on the Rights of the Child, 1959/1989
- UN Convention on the Rights of People with Disabilities, 2006
- *Quality and Fairness – A Health System for You*, 2001
- *A Vision for Change – Report of the Expert Group on Mental Health Policy*, 2006
- National Policy on Children and Young People in Ireland, 2000
- *Traveller Health – A National Strategy 2002–2005*.

There are numerous other policies, and when working in a specialist area staff will identify the legislation and policies relevant to their field of practice. Organisations are also expected to write their own policies that work in line with national legislation and policy. Before commencing work with any organisation, staff will be given organisational policies that must be read and adhered to.

Due to the lack of awareness relating to policies, in 1994 the then Minister for Health, Brendan Howlin, published the health policy document *Shaping a Healthier Future*. He ensured that all people working within the then Health Boards, no matter what their role, would know about the new policy. It was printed in a colourful, easy-to-read format and every staff member – doctors, nurses, care staff, physiotherapists as well as cooks, cleaners and porters – were expected to attend an information session and a copy of the policy was given to each staff member.

Task

Compare copies of the following health policies: *Health: The Wider Dimensions* (1986) and *Shaping a Healthier Future* (1994). You will see how the different presentation of the 1994 policy made it more accessible. Look at a copy of the current policy, *Quality and Fairness – A Health System for You* (2001).

STATUTORY AND VOLUNTARY ORGANISATIONS

In Ireland, health care is delivered through a public/private mix. While there is ongoing debate around the issues relating to this model, it is sufficient for students to know the differences between the different types of organisations: statutory, voluntary and private.

Statutory bodies are those that are established and funded by the state (in the case of health care, through the Department of Health).

Voluntary organisations are those that are usually established locally to meet the needs of a specific target group, for example the Irish Wheelchair Association and the Multiple Sclerosis Society. These organisations are usually funded through voluntary donations and fundraising events, with small grants often made available from the Department of Health. However, many larger organisations, particularly religious organisations, have established hospitals and community support services and receive a substantial proportion of their funding from the state while still retaining their voluntary status, for example the Brothers of Charity services for people with intellectual disabilities, the Mater Hospital and St Vincent's Hospital. The 1994 health strategy, *Shaping a Healthier Future*, is underpinned by the principles of equity, quality of service and accountability, and while it acknowledged the work of the voluntary organisations and agreed that 'the independent identity of voluntary agencies will be fully respected', it also insisted for the first time that the organisations were to be accountable to the health authorities for the public funds that they received from them (Department of Health 1994: 33).

Services delivered through private practice include GP services and many private residential and nursing homes for older people. *Shaping a Healthier Future* suggested that appropriate monitoring and consultative mechanisms should be established involving the Department of Health, the public health services and the institutional providers of private care to address a number of relevant issues, including examining the processes in place in private hospitals for the maintenance of acceptable standards and good practice and the review of complaints made by or on behalf of patients (Department of Health 1994: 37).

HIQA

The Health Information and Quality Authority (HIQA) is an independent authority established in May 2007 to drive continuous improvement in Ireland's health and social care services. This is probably the organisation that most care staff will hear about, so it is important that all CCAs know and understand HIQA's roles and responsibilities, particularly in their own area of practice. There is a short summary of them below.

Reporting directly to the Minister for Health, HIQA's role is to promote quality and safety in the provision of health and personal social services for the benefit of the health and welfare of the public.

As an independent organisation, HIQA is committed to an open and transparent relationship with its stakeholders. Their independence within the health system is fundamental to their functional success.

Their mandate extends across the quality and safety of the public, private (within their social care function) and voluntary sectors. It also has statutory responsibility for the following.

* **Setting standards for health and social services:** Developing the quality and safety standards, based on evidence and best international practice, for health and social care services in Ireland (except mental health services).

* **Monitoring health care quality:** Monitoring standards of quality and safety in the health services and investigating serious concerns about the health and welfare of service users as necessary.

* **Health technology assessment:** Ensuring the best outcome for the service user by evaluating the clinical and economic effectiveness of drugs, equipment, diagnostic techniques and health promotion activities.

* **Health information:** Advising on the collection and sharing of information across the services, evaluating information and publishing information about the delivery and performance of Ireland's health and social care services.

* **Social Services Inspectorate:** Registration and inspection of residential homes for children, older people and people with disabilities where applicable. Monitoring day and pre-school facilities and children's detention centres and inspecting foster care services. During 2009, HIQA continued to maintain its momentum in undertaking its core functions and also commenced a new statutory function. From 1 July 2009, HIQA assumed responsibility for the registration and inspection of all residential care services for older people. For the first time, centres run by the HSE as well as private and voluntary nursing homes were subject to independent registration and inspection (www.hiqa.ie, 11 July 2012).

HIQA is responsible for introducing the minimum qualification of FETAC level 5 for all care assistants working in residential care settings for older people (standard 24.2).

Task

Download the HIQA standards relevant to your area of work. Read them carefully and consider how they are implemented in your workplace.

MODELS OF HEALTH

Because health care is so broad, there is a need to identify the relevant frameworks for working as a CCA so that you are both equipped and supported in care practice. The following models, theories and frameworks will help to clarify the differences between the models and dimensions of health and provide a firm structure to base care practice on.

It is important to understand that the social and medical models of health complement rather than compete with each other, although there is often tension and competition relating to funding, resources and professional pride. As mentioned already, the focus of the medical model is 'treat and cure'. This applies to a wide range of acute or chronic illnesses, from common colds and flu that may need symptomatic relief with over-the-counter medication, e.g. Paracetamol and Lemsip, to more severe infections that may need antibiotics, to acute medical emergencies that may need surgical interventions, e.g. appendicitis, fractured limbs. Sometimes a person with a disability may develop an infection or medical emergency that needs to be treated with medication or in an acute hospital setting, while others may have two or more conditions that need simultaneous interventions from within the medical and social model of health.

DIMENSIONS OF HEALTH

It is difficult to make absolute distinctions between the dimensions or models of health because there is often an overlap, but it is important to understand where each can be applied in practice.

Ewles and Simnett (2003) identified six dimensions of health, as listed below. However, others have identified a greater or lesser number and it will be noticeable that there are strong links between the dimensions. For example, Ewles and Simnett cite sexual health as crossing all of the dimensions (Ewles and Simnett 2003: 7). This is a particularly useful framework for assessing and understanding the range of a client's needs.

Physical health

This is perhaps the most obvious dimension of health and is concerned with the mechanistic functioning of the body.

Mental health

Mental health means the ability to think clearly and coherently. This is distinct from emotional and social health, although the three are closely associated.

Emotional health

This means the ability to recognise emotions such as fear, joy, grief and anger and to express such emotions appropriately. Emotional health (sometimes called affective health) also means coping with stress, tension, depression and anxiety.

Social health

Social health means the ability to make and maintain relationships with other people.

Spiritual health

For some people, spiritual health is connected with religious beliefs and practices, while for other people it is to do with personal creeds, principles of behaviour and ways of achieving peace of mind and being at peace with oneself.

Societal health

So far health has been considered at an individual level, but a person's health is inextricably related to everything surrounding that person. It is impossible to be healthy in a 'sick' society that doesn't provide the resources for basic physical and emotional needs. For example, people obviously can't be healthy if they can't afford the necessities for food, clothing and shelter, but neither can they be healthy in countries of extreme political oppression where basic human rights are denied. Women can't be healthy when their contribution to society is undervalued, and neither black nor white people can be healthy in a society where racism undermines human worth, self-esteem and social relationships. Unemployed people can't be healthy in a society that only values people in paid employment, and it is very unlikely that anyone can be healthy if they live in an area that lacks basic services and facilities such as health care, transport and recreation (Ewles and Simnett 2003: 6).

A HOLISTIC PERSPECTIVE OF HEALTH

Over the years, the World Health Organisation (WHO) has defined health in a number of ways. Their 1948 Constitution stipulated:

Health is a state of complete physical, mental and social well-being and not merely the absence of disease or infirmity.

However, this definition was criticised for being unrealistic and simplistic. It is argued that no individual can meet these requirements for any length of time. Furthermore, it implies that health remains static, whereas we know that an individual's health status fluctuates regularly. A more recent definition addresses these points and clarifies health as:

The extent to which an individual or group is able to realise aspirations and satisfy needs and to change or cope with the environment. Health is a resource for everyday life, not the object of living; it is a positive concept, emphasising social and personal resources as well as physical capabilities. (WHO 1984)

In England during the 1970s there was growing concern about the inequalities in the health status of different groups of people. A famous review was undertaken and a report, the Black report, was published in 1980. This report identified a number of determinants of health, including social class, occupation, gender, economic conditions and geographical location. It recognised the differences in the health status of people in relation to nutrition, education, housing, unemployment, reduced social support network and stress, with poorer people being more disadvantaged than wealthier people. The Economic and Social Research Institute (ESRI) is a not-for-profit organisation that undertakes independent research in Ireland relating to issues such as poverty and health.

People who need care can be grouped by age, gender, ethnicity or disability, for example children, adolescents, older people, women, men, Travellers, refugees/asylum seekers, people with mental health difficulties, people with physical disabilities, people with learning difficulties or unemployed people. There can be further grouping according to a specific disability or ethnicity, for example older people with Down syndrome, children with autism, adolescents with mental health difficulties, unemployed men with mental health difficulties and women Travellers. When a person can be grouped into two or more categories, there are two or more disadvantages to live with and this usually compounds their health difficulties, which reduces their health status.

Therefore, a holistic perspective of health is most relevant in health care today. Such care encompasses the whole person and does not focus on the disability or illness in isolation. If somebody has to undergo major treatment or surgery that will keep them out of work or away from home for some time, there is anxiety around surgery and hospitalisation, but also social stresses and anxieties – for example, who will care for the children? pay the mortgage? buy the food? drive the car? walk and feed the dog? The result of not delivering holistic care may mean that the patient will not have enough time to fully recuperate and will return to work or caring responsibilities or doing household chores too soon, which in turn slows down full recovery or precipitates a relapse. This situation can be compounded if the needs of the individual are more long term or permanent, as with a person with a disability or a member of an ethnic minority group.

In addition, issues such as those identified in the Black report are all stressors that quite often lead to behaviours that are detrimental to health, for example smoking, poor diet and lack of exercise, which in turn leads to a reduction in mental health status and well-being as well as physical illnesses such as coronary heart disease, strokes and cancers. The recognition and acceptance of these facts, after some initial resistance to the ideas, created the foundations of the health promotion movement in the 1970s.

In 1984, WHO defined health promotion as:

The process of enabling people to increase control over, and to improve, their health.

This definition was in line with the more recent WHO definition of health, and in 1986 the first health promotion conference was held in Ottawa, Canada. During this conference, ways in which this definition could be activated or realised were identified and they constitute the five principles of health promotion. These principles are known as the Ottawa Charter:

- Building healthy public policy
- Creating supportive environments
- Developing personal skills through information and education in health and life skills
- Strengthening community participation
- Reorienting health services towards the prevention of illness and disease towards health promotion

This charter clearly demonstrated that health should be looked at positively rather than negatively, i.e. in relation to sickness. There was an attempt to divert responsibility for health away from the medical teams of doctors and nurses and towards individuals, communities and local authorities. This charter acknowledged that people would need support with this change of focus and it included personal resources, public policy and health education in the remit.

In 1990, Downie, Tannahill and Tannahill developed a model of health promotion that identified three overlapping spheres and seven domains for achieving this (see Figure 1.1).

Figure 1.1: Downie, Tannahill and Tannahill's model of health promotion

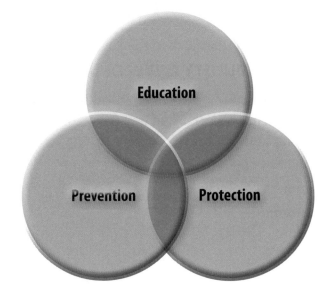

Source: Downie, Tannahill and Tannahill (1990).

◆ **Health education**, such as community education programmes and health promotion strategies incorporated within the primary and secondary school curriculum taught by teachers rather than visiting nurses.

◆ **Protection**, such as wearing cycle helmets, seat belts and using car seats for children, smoking ban in public places.

◆ **Prevention**, such as vaccination programmes and the fluoridation of water, although these issues are contentious at times and need wider debate. Strategies aimed at raising public awareness relating to the health risks associated with alcohol and tobacco try to reduce the number of people who engage in risky behaviours.

Since the 1970s there have been many advances in the field of health promotion. CCAs will find themselves incorporating health promotion strategies into their care practice almost automatically, but it is necessary to consider the importance of planned approaches for people in receipt of care.

Task

Identify three health promotion strategies that you incorporate into your daily life. Are the same strategies relevant to the people in your care?

PRINCIPLES OF COMMUNITY DEVELOPMENT

Community development can be viewed as a health promotion strategy with closely connected principles working at the same three levels of personal, community and policy and working towards:

◆ Social justice
◆ Self-determination
◆ Sustainable communities
◆ Participation
◆ Equality
◆ Empowerment.

There are a number of support services and resources for people in the community, funded and delivered through the Departments of Health and Social Protection as well as voluntary organisations, for example family support services, Traveller training programmes, and programmes for early school leavers, lone parents and people with disabilities. It is important that CCAs are aware of the community development supports and services that are available in their locality so as to strengthen the opportunities available to people in receipt of care.

MASLOW'S HIERARCHY OF NEEDS

Humanistic psychology is a branch of psychology that developed in the 1950s and 60s in response to what was seen as negative beliefs about behaviour that underpinned other types of psychology. Well-known humanistic psychologists such as Abraham Maslow (1908–70) and Carl Rogers (1902–87) argued that people are not trapped by their earlier unconscious experiences, instinct or environment, but have a great ability to utilise their internal resources of feelings, values and hope to take control of their own lives, regardless of their age or circumstances. Again, this is an area worthy of further study, but in this chapter we will consider a theory that was developed by Maslow in 1943 – Maslow's hierarchy of needs. Maslow suggests that there is an order of needs that motivates human behaviour and that a person must meet their basic needs before they can move on to higher needs. The pyramid shape is used to illustrate these needs, with the greater needs at the bottom, wider part of the pyramid. The needs are grouped as physiological, safety, social, esteem and self-actualisation.

Figure 1.2: Maslow's hierarchy of needs

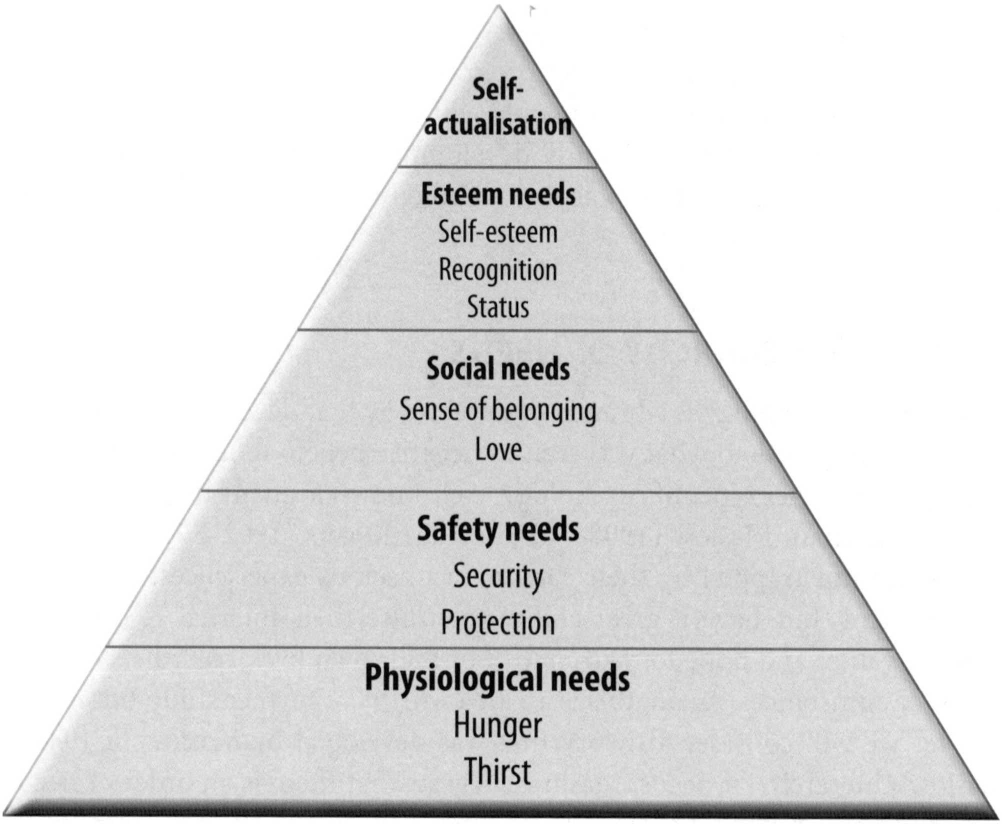

Source: Maslow (1970).

Physiological needs

This need is associated with the essentials that we need to survive: food, water, air, sleep. If we do not have these basics, we can't move on to the next level.

Safety needs

Once physiological needs are met, then the individual can move on to the next level of safety and security. People who are starving are prepared to compromise their safety in order to get food, but once they are no longer hungry, they can turn their attention to shelter. This means more than (but can start with) shelter from the environmental elements – it includes a safe neighbourhood, the security of employment, a regular supply of food and adequate health care, including protection from illness (as in vaccination programmes).

Social needs

Humans have a need to love and be loved. Relationships are very important and there is a need for acceptance, belonging, love or affection. Belonging to or being affiliated with a family, a community or a religious organisation can meet those needs.

Esteem needs

Self-esteem is about having regard for, valuing and accepting the person you are. It is about the need for competence and the ability to achieve what you set out to do as well as to gain recognition and approval.

Self-actualisation

According to Maslow, this is the peak experience – to find self-fulfilment by realising your full potential. However, he also suggested that people who achieve self-actualisation do not reach it and do nothing else; they always set themselves new challenges and so push themselves to achieve more.

ERIKSON'S DEVELOPMENTAL STAGES

Erik Erikson (1902–94) developed a theory of lifelong psycho-social development that involves eight stages during a lifespan. As with previous theories, this theory should be studied in greater depth, but for the purposes of this chapter it will be considered as a way of understanding the needs of the people you will be working with.

Table 1.1: Erikson's developmental stages

Stage	Basic conflict	Important events	Outcome
Infancy (birth to 18 months)	Trust vs. mistrust	Feeding	Children develop a sense of trust when caregivers provide reliability, care and affection. A lack of this will lead to mistrust.
Early childhood (2–3 years)	Autonomy vs. shame and doubt	Toilet training	Children need to develop a sense of personal control over physical skills and a sense of independence. Success leads to feelings of autonomy, while failure results in feelings of shame and doubt.
Preschool (3–5 years)	Initiative vs. guilt	Exploration	Children need to begin asserting control and power over the environment. Success in this stage leads to a sense of purpose. Children who try to exert too much power experience disapproval, resulting in a sense of guilt.
School age (6–11 years)	Industry vs. inferiority	School	Children need to cope with new social and academic demands. Success leads to a sense of competence, while failure results in feelings of inferiority.
Adolescence (12–18 years)	Identity vs. role confusion	Social relationships	Teens need to develop a sense of self and personal identity. Success leads to an ability to stay true to yourself, while failure leads to role confusion and a weak sense of self.
Young adulthood (19–40 years)	Intimacy vs. isolation	Relationships	Young adults need to form intimate, loving relationships with other people. Success leads to strong relationships, while failure results in loneliness and isolation.
Middle adulthood (40–65 years)	Generativity vs. stagnation	Work and parenthood	Adults need to create or nurture things that will outlast them, often by having children or creating a positive change that benefits other people. Success leads to feelings of usefulness and accomplishment, while failure results in shallow involvement in the world.
Maturity (65 to death)	Ego integrity vs. despair	Reflection on life	Older adults need to look back on life and feel a sense of fulfilment. Success at this stage leads to feelings of wisdom, while failure results in regret, bitterness and despair.

Erikson argued that people have an ability to develop across their lifespan and that early childhood experiences do not permanently shape personality. As can be seen in Table 1.1, at each stage there is a crisis or conflict that needs to be balanced before resolution and movement to the next stage. The key lies in balance rather than emphasis on either extreme. For example, although people need to learn to trust the world and others, they also need to maintain some mistrust to protect them from danger. For people with chronic illnesses or disabilities, these stages of development will be different; they may be delayed or impaired and their disability will influence their development. This theory of development continues until death, which is why it is important for CCAs who are delivering end-of-life care to appreciate the importance of it.

Task

Can you understand the application of Erikson's stages of lifelong development in relation to the people you are caring for?

This section of the chapter has identified a number of structures that are embedded within care practice, and while legislation and policy must be strictly adhered to, models and theories are used as looser frameworks for care and elements of each can be used in different situations or circumstances. You can probably identify the overlaps between the different models and theories and understand the broader context of health and how an understanding of the frameworks will support you in your work.

CARE PROVISION

When thinking about care provision, one of the first questions we could ask is who needs care. Sometimes it is easy to recognise individuals or groups of people who need care, while at other times those in need are less visible. Furthermore, there is a need to develop a clearer understanding of the conditions and related issues that arise for different groups of people.

Also included in the list below are children (young people up to the age of 18) and women.

Disability

Under the Disability Act 2005, the term 'disability' in relation to a person is defined as:

a substantial restriction in the capacity of the person to carry on a profession, business or occupation in the State or to participate in social or cultural life in the State by reason of an enduring physical, sensory, mental health or intellectual impairment. (Part 1, section 2, page 6)

Further, 'assessment' means:

an assessment undertaken or arranged by the Executive to determine, in respect of a person with a disability, the health and education needs (if any) occasioned by the disability and the health services or education services (if any) required to meet those needs. (Part 2, section 7, page 9)

Culture

This is a society or group's total way of life, including customs, traditions, beliefs, values, language and physical products, from tools to artwork – all learned behaviour passed from parents to children. Culture is not static; it is constantly changing, often with contact from other cultures.

Ethnicity

An ethnic group consists of people united by ancestry, race, religion, language and/or national origin, which contribute to a sense of shared identity and shared attitudes, beliefs and values. Most ethnic groups trace their roots to a country of origin.

Travellers

Travellers are an indigenous minority ethnic group who date back for some centuries. According to the 2011 census, there are approximately 24,500 Travellers living in Ireland. They have their own set of traditions, values, culture and language. The inequalities and poor health status of Travellers are well documented.

Refugees/asylum seekers

A refugee is a person who has had to leave their country because of war, natural disaster or persecution on the grounds of race, religion, political opinion or social group. Refugees who have to wait in a country and apply for residency there are called asylum seekers.

Older people

With life expectancy growing and the retirement age increasing, old age has been classified in developed countries as early old age (65–75 years), middle old age (75–85 years) and very old age (over 85 years).

CONDITIONS ASSOCIATED WITH DISABILITY

It is important for CCAs to know and understand the conditions that affect the people in their care. Included here is a short list of conditions associated with disability. It is not exhaustive but it demonstrates how each condition is classified. Sometimes one condition can be classified in two sections, for example cerebral palsy.

Physical disabilities

- Acquired brain injury
- Cerebral palsy
- Conditions associated with systems, e.g. circulatory/respiratory/lymphatic, asthma/epilepsy/diabetes
- Motor neurone disease
- Multiple sclerosis
- Muscular dystrophy
- Spinal injury
- Stroke

Learning disabilities

- Asperger syndrome
- Autism
- Cerebral palsy
- Challenging behaviour

+ Down syndrome
+ Other genetic conditions, including Williams, Rett, Prader-Willi and fragile X syndromes

Mental health difficulties

+ Addictions, e.g. drugs, alcohol
+ Bipolar disorder
+ Dementia
+ Depression
+ Eating disorders
+ Obsessive compulsive disorder (OCD)
+ Post-traumatic stress disorder (PTSD)
+ Post-natal depression
+ Schizophrenia
+ Suicidal thoughts and behaviours

Different types of care are needed by people with different conditions and needs. For example, a person with motor neurone disease may need to be washed, dressed and fed, while a person with chronic depression or a mild learning disability may need prompting to wash, dress and eat.

Task

Can you differentiate between the different types of disability? Think about the people in your care – can you identify their conditions or disabilities?

WHAT DO WE CALL PEOPLE WHO RECEIVE CARE SERVICES?

Traditionally in care practice, everybody was called a 'patient', reflecting the medical model and the 'sick role'. In recent years within the social model of health, people using services and their families have been involved in discussions about all aspects of their care, and that includes how they would like to be addressed. *Vision for Change* (2007), the expert report on mental health services, and Inclusion Ireland, the National Association for People with an

Intellectual Disability, arrived at two different titles – 'service user' and 'person' or 'individual' – reflecting the individuality between groups. Other terms include 'client', 'resident' or 'case'. In this text we will use the terms 'individual' or 'person'.

CARE PRACTICE

As discussed earlier, care can be delivered through community development projects and support systems or through health care organisations. The different types of care needs will be met by different professional practitioners. In this section, attention will be focused on care for people who need assistance and support in the activities of daily living (ADLs).

CCAs are usually employed to assist and support people with their ADLs. Traditionally, health care was task focused and related to what the health care professional did to or for the patient. A strict routine was in place and the patient was a passive recipient of care, while the professionals were the experts who knew what was best, often delivering 'one size fits all' care. People were often woken up in the very early hours of the morning and put back to bed in the middle of the afternoon with no stimulation or entertainment during the day in order to accommodate staff work rotas.

Fundamental to the social model of health has been the emphasis on person-centred care, whereby each individual will have a specific care plan so that their needs always take priority in care practice. The therapeutic benefits of leisure and activity to health and well-being have been well documented and these are included in the care plan.

There are numerous reasons why an individual will need care. In setting the standards for social care services, HIQA (2009) has laid out the principles that underpin social care practice as being:

* Open and transparent
* Focused on outcomes
* Person centred
* Evidence based.

Whether assisting a client or performing a task for a client, there are a number of basic premises.

- **Permission:** Always explain what you are going to do and check that the client understands and consents.

- **Privacy:** Ensure that there is privacy by taking the client to a bedroom or bathroom where they will not be observed or overheard by other people. Be discreet when bathing, showering and toileting a client.

- **Promote independence:** Sometimes there is an urge to carry out the task for the client, as they may find it difficult or awkward, but the CCA's role is to encourage, support and advise if necessary. It may take a little longer or be less efficient, but clients are entitled to their independence.

- **Confidentiality:** Do not discuss the client or related information with anyone other than the client and the MDT. As a CCA it is usually best to refer requests for information to your line manager. The client must always consent to information being divulged to a third party.

In order to comply with these principles there must be a structured method for planning care. This is achieved initially by using a formal process, like the nursing process. This is a framework that can be used in social care as well as acute nursing and is an alternative to the traditional task-orientated approach to care practice. There are five cyclical elements to the nursing process – assessment, diagnosis, planning, implementation and evaluation – and it is important that all members of the MDT adhere to this process to ensure quality care for the individual.

Figure 1.3: The stages of the nursing process

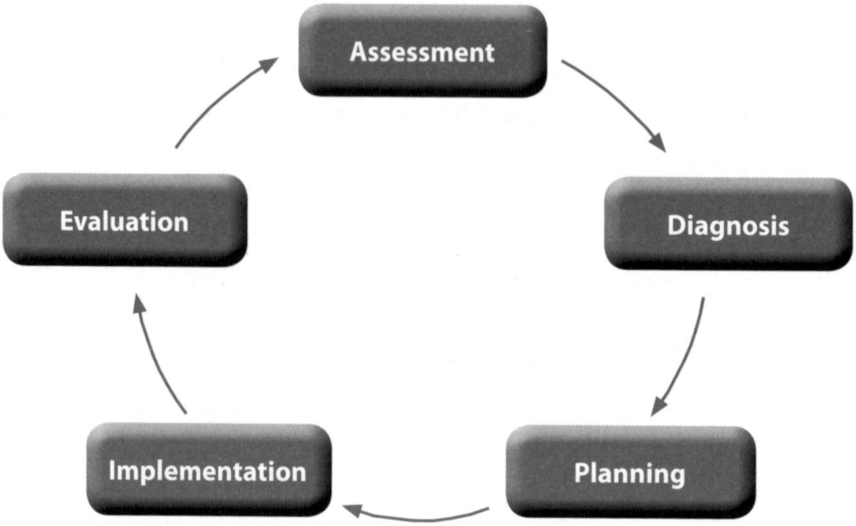

Assessment

Diagnosis

Planning

Implementation

Evaluation

The first stage of the process is an assessment of the individual's needs based on information collated from the client, the family, GP and PHN and medical and nursing records. Assessments are carried out by a member of the MDT, usually a nurse, PHN, OT or manager of a unit, depending on whether the person is in hospital, residential care or living in the community. Again, there is a process involved in assessments to ensure standardisation and a number of assessment tools have been developed over the years, for example the Katz index, the Barthel index and the Roper, Logan, Tierney model of nursing assessment. However, many organisations will devise their own specific index. Whichever tool is used, their purpose is to assess a client's ability and independence within the ADLs and a care plan is devised on the basis of this assessment. For example:

+ **Breathing:** Any acute or chronic respiratory illness, cough, sputum, smoking history.
+ **Communication:** Vision, hearing, speech, comprehension.
+ **Controlling body temperature:** Pyrexia/hypothermia, feels cold/heat.
+ **Dying:** Fears expressed, wishes, sacrament of the sick.
+ **Eating and drinking:** Appetite, therapeutic diet, food allergies, assistance with dietary intake, swallowing, gut function.
+ **Eliminating:** Continent of urine, diarrhoea/constipation, strain/difficulty/pain on defecation, effects of food/medication on bowel function, recent changes in bowel habit.
+ **Expressing sexuality:** Sexual history, body image, gender-related beliefs, roles, practices.
+ **Maintenance of a safe environment:** Memory, orientation to time, place, person, history of falls, risk of infection, risk of abuse, balance between well-being and safety issues.
+ **Mobility:** Level of independence, getting in/out of bed, moving around house/unit, repositioning in chair, walking outside.
+ **Pain:** Type of pain, if any.
+ **Personal and oral hygiene:** Condition of mouth, dentures, skin, hair, nails, needs assistance, independent.
+ **Sleeping:** Sleeping pattern, sedation, night routine.
+ **Working and playing:** Work, home and leisure activities, daily routine, exercise, family commitments, social networks.

Although the ADLs mostly relate to physical aspects of health, reduced capacity in any of these areas will impact other dimensions, as can be seen in the list below. Individual needs can also be linked to Maslow's hierarchy of needs and Erikson's stages of development to ensure that all aspects of health are included to assist a person in achieving their potential in line with their stage of development.

This list can be studied, discussed and extended. For example, loss of appetite can be caused by physical reasons but may also impact on the other dimensions – even spiritual health is included here because eating and drinking play a large part in people's spiritual lives, either because of associated food preparation, fasting or feasting rituals.

- **Breathing:** Physical, mental, emotional and social.
- **Communication:** Physical, mental, emotional and social.
- **Controlling body temperature:** Physical, mental, social and societal.
- **Dying:** Physical, mental, emotional, social, spiritual and societal.
- **Eating and drinking:** Physical, mental, emotional, social, spiritual and societal.
- **Eliminating:** Physical, emotional, social.
- **Expressing sexuality:** Physical, mental, emotional, social, spiritual and societal.
- **Maintenance of a safe environment:** Physical, mental and societal.
- **Mobility:** Physical, mental, emotional, social, spiritual and societal.
- **Pain:** Physical, mental, emotional, social, spiritual and societal.
- **Personal and oral hygiene:** Physical, mental, emotional, social and societal.
- **Sleeping:** Physical, emotional and social.
- **Working and playing:** Physical, mental, emotional, social, spiritual and societal.

Task

Access one type of index, either via the internet or through your workplace setting.

The second part of the nursing process – diagnosis – is the remit of medical staff, but it is important for the CCA to know and understand the diagnosis in order to anticipate the needs of the individual that are associated with the condition.

Once the diagnosis has been made a person-centred care plan will be drawn up. As with assessments, care plans are usually drawn up by a member of the MDT, usually the person who has carried out the assessment. Care plans are based on:

+ Dignity and respect
+ Empowerment
+ Choices
+ Rights.

The care plan is discussed with the client as well as the MDT and is a practical way of communicating information accurately within the MDT. Furthermore, new staff can access client history without asking repetitive questions of the client and their family. Ideally, the care plan will:

+ Summarise the client's health status, issues and goals
+ Indicate personal preferences
+ Suggest a daily routine
+ Contain contact details for key workers and next of kin
+ Contain review dates.

Copies of the care plan will be kept by the individual and their CCAs and they are examined during a HIQA inspection. Confidentiality and consent are priorities in relation to client information.

The fourth stage of the nursing process – implementation – is of major importance to the CCA, as they are responsible for delivering practical care. CCAs must be fully informed as to the assessment and the care plan for each client and the care plan must be consulted and fully implemented. Short-term and long-term goals are included in the care plan and any new information accessed or any changes in the condition of the individual must be reported to the line manager and documented. If necessary, an earlier evaluation is carried out and changes in the care plan can be made. Otherwise, a full evaluation is carried out within the original timeframe and the process begins again.

Task

Take the list of ADLs and create lists that relate to Maslow's hierarchy of needs and Erikson's stages of development.

SUMMARY

Two aspects of care have been explored in this chapter: care provision and practice. Within these aspects there is an array of topics that need careful consideration, including the people who need care, models of health and health promotion, theories and structures upon which to base care practice as well as an outline of the legislation and policies that govern it. A good knowledge and understanding of this module will provide the foundation for the delivery of high-quality, holistic care.

REFERENCES

Department of Health (1994) *Shaping a Healthier Future: A Strategy for Effective Healthcare in the 1990s*, Dublin: Stationery Office.

Department of Health and Children (2005) Disability Act 2005, Dublin: Stationery Office.

Downie, R.S., Tannahill, C. and Tannahill, A. (1990) *Health Promotion: Models and Values*, Oxford: Oxford University Press.

Ewles, L. and Simnett, I. (2003) *Promoting Health – A Practical Guide*, 5th edition, London: Balliere Tindall.

HIQA (2009) *National Quality Standards: Residential Services for People with Disabilities*, Cork: HIQA.

Maslow, A.H. (1970) *Motivation and Personality*, 2nd edition, New York: Harper & Row.

Papalia, D.E., Wendkos Olds, S. and Duskin Feldman, R. (2001) *Human Development*, 8th international edition, New York: McGraw-Hill.

WHO (1984), *Health Promotion: A Discussion Document*, Copenhagen: WHO.

2
Understanding Ageing

INTRODUCTION

This chapter explores the concept of ageing and the potential to promote healthy ageing through good care supporting individuals across all the dimensions of health. Attitudes to ageing will be explored and holistic ways to enhance the quality of life of older people will be considered. Throughout the text, you will discover ways to implement best practice in your care setting.

KEY TERMS

- advocacy
- cognitive
- empathy
- empowerment
- health promotion
- HIQA
- impaired
- independence
- mobility
- multidisciplinary
- sensory

UNDERSTANDING AGEING

According to the World Health Organisation (WHO), in the next few years there will be more people in the world aged over 60 than children aged less than five for the first time. At its World Heath Day in 2012, the WHO called for 'urgent action to ensure that, at a time when the world's population is ageing rapidly, people reach old age in the best possible health'.

Our first objective is to define 'age'. The ageing process is, of course, a biological reality with its own dynamic; this is largely beyond human control.

However, it is also subject to the constructions through which each society makes sense of age. In developed nations, for example, chronological time plays a paramount role and age 60 to 65 is considered to be the beginning of old age. It must be borne in mind that this is a social construct. In other words, we as a society 'construct' how we view ageing. It is important to differentiate between ageing and healthy ageing because, as with younger people, the ageing person's health and welfare will be affected by illness, whether it is physical, psychological or social in nature.

Task

Can you think of reasons why countries need to balance their birth rate with their ageing population?

We face a major challenge in society today. Our rapidly ageing society will bring with it difficulties associated with ageing, such as physical infirmity, nervous system disorders and sensory loss, which all increase with age. On the other hand, there has never been a better time to be old. People are experiencing healthy longevity as never before in the history of mankind.

AGEING IN IRELAND

We have one of the lowest proportions of population aged over 65 in the European Union. The 2011 census shows Ireland's population of older people aged 65 and over to be at 535,393. Our population is slowly ageing and it is estimated that by 2041, 22% of the population will be over the age of 65 years. In Ireland we are fortunate that we also have one of the highest birth rates in the European Union.

Services for older people in Ireland

The Health Service Executive (HSE) provides a wide range of services for people growing older in Ireland. Supports are also available from other agencies, such as the Department of Social Protection, local authorities and voluntary organisations.

The Nursing Homes Support Scheme can support older people who require long-term nursing home care. This scheme is better known as the 'Fair Deal'. Under this scheme the person will make a contribution towards the cost of care and the state will meet the cost of the balance. This scheme is available to use in public, private and voluntary nursing homes.

Older people in Ireland are entitled to a range of benefits and schemes to help with medical costs and daily living. Everyone over the age of 66 in Ireland is entitled to a state pension, either contributory or non-contributory. Currently, every person aged over 70 is entitled to a Medical Card and will benefit from the Drug Payment Scheme. All individuals are entitled to be assessed to avail of Home Care Packages. Other benefits include optical benefits, hearing aid grants, respite care grants and the Community Support for Older People Scheme. The HSE has responsibility for the protection of older people from elder abuse.

Older people in Ireland are also supported through voluntary agencies, such as Age Action, that offer a range of information services and supports to older people. Agencies such as the Alzheimer's Society of Ireland offer support to people who suffer from this disease and their families. People with this illness are increasingly being supported through private home care provision.

The Health Information and Equality Authority (HIQA) was established as a result of the implementation of the Health Act 2007. Its remit is to drive improvements in the quality and safety of health care on behalf of patients. HIQA began inspecting residential services for older people in 2009. It makes recommendations following inspection, where necessary, and all reports are available on its website (www.hiqa.ie). According to HIQA:

These quality standards were developed based on legislation, research findings and best practice. They were developed in partnership with service users, service providers, health care professionals, older people's representative groups, the Department of Health and Children and the Health Service Executive.

Currently, older people in Ireland avail of health services through their GP and public health nurse. It has been proposed for some years that primary care services would be supported by a primary care team. The objective of primary care teams is to circumvent hospital admission (known as 'secondary care') through the primary supports offered through a multidisciplinary team. Unfortunately, the roll-out of this service has been poor and patchy. Additionally, many posts are vacant due to the HSE's moratorium on recruitment. It is hoped that in the future these teams will fully develop, creating stronger supports for older people living in the community.

A multidisciplinary team (MDT) should consist of a:

- GP
- Public health nurse
- Occupational therapist
- Physiotherapist
- Psychologist
- Social worker
- Home care team

THE AGEING PROCESS

There are some biological changes that can occur as we get older. However, these are individualised and differ from person to person according to lifestyle and history. Growing old is something that happens to us all. Although we may not all experience disease or chronic illness as we age, almost all of us will lose some form of 'function' as we age.

Task

How do you think positive, healthy ageing can be promoted?

Ageing is influenced by all of the following.

Figure 2.1: Influences on ageing

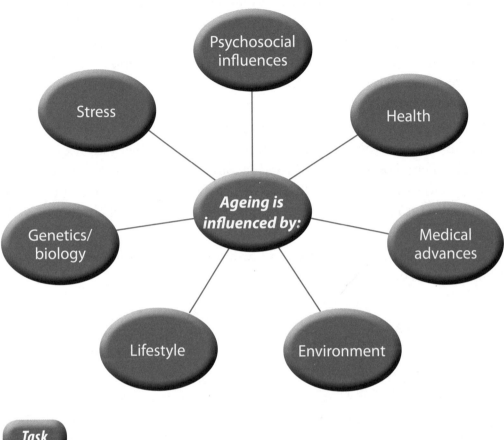

Task

Referring to the previous headings, consider how you think these factors influence ageing.

According to Tyas et al (2007), 'Healthy ageing encompasses health in its broadest sense, with the quality of life maintained or enhanced into older age.' In our advancing years it is important to remain engaged and active in society. Organisations such as Age Action Ireland play a pivotal role in supporting the ageing population through the organisation of activities. As we live in a work-orientated society, retirement may mean people experience:

- Loss of social contact through work
- Loss of their 'sense of purpose'
- Loss of status.

The process of engaging older people as they age can become more difficult due to the development of age-related disabilities. Individual, community, public and private sector approaches are required to promote the health of individuals in the ageing population. Such approaches will aim to maintain and improve the physical, emotional and social well-being of older people. HIQA standard 12 requires that all residential services for older people will promote the health of those in their care.

It is important that society can support individuals in preparing for retirement so that the mental, physical and social changes are experienced gradually. Planning for life on a fixed income is essential, as low income has an impact on the overall health and well-being of all individuals in society, affecting everything from physical health status to social and emotional well-being.

As we age, changes may occur in our body. Below is a list of some of the common areas of decline as we age.

Body appearance

+ **Skin:** Skin is the largest organ in the body, protecting the body from disease and infection. The skin loses some of its elasticity as we age, which makes it more vulnerable to damage. Ageing skin can also make an older person more vulnerable to pressure ulcers. As we age, there may be reduced blood flow to the skin and the amount of fat under the skin tends to decrease as people get older.

+ **Nails:** Nails grow more slowly and can become thicker and more difficult to cut and maintain.

+ **Hair:** Both men and women may suffer from hair loss and hair may turn grey. Some women grow facial hair after the menopause due to a change in hormone levels.

Body movement

+ **Muscles:** Older people are at particular risk of muscle weakness and a reduction in mobility. It is very important to remain active in order to maximise muscle strength, maintain co-ordination and reduce the risk of falls.

• **Joints and bones:** Osteoarthritis is characterised by the destruction of cartilage, which usually affects weight-bearing joints, e.g. knees and hips. It commonly occurs in older people as joints wear out. Osteoarthritis is more common in females and obesity increases the risk. Joints affected can include shoulder, hip, knees, hands and spine. Cartilage between joints becomes worn away, making movements painful and difficult (Byrnes 2011). Older people may develop a stoop caused by a curve in the spine, which may reduce the person's height by several centimetres. Osteoporosis is caused by a lack of calcium, making bones light and brittle. It affects one in two women and one in five men. People who develop osteoporosis fracture their bones very easily. Twenty per cent of people over the age of 60 who fracture a hip can die within six to 12 months. It is essential to protect older people from falls through careful management and monitoring of their environment, particularly if they suffer from osteoarthritis or osteoporosis.

The circulatory system

Cardiovascular disease can occur as a result of diseased arteries, which supply blood to the heart and other parts of the body. They become blocked and eventually the blood supply is cut off, which can lead to a heart attack or stroke. Cardiovascular disease can be due to genetics and is more common in men. People with higher risk factors include those who smoke, have high blood pressure, have higher levels of cholesterol, have diabetes, have a poor diet, are obese or lead an inactive lifestyle. Bacterial and viral infections can play a role in the development of cardiovascular disease, which is the leading cause of death worldwide (Byrnes 2011: 76).

Older people may develop heart failure. This can be for a range of reasons, but again, the risk factors for this disease are linked to lifestyle. Heart failure occurs when the heart cannot pump as it should to meet the needs of the body.

The respiratory system

The lungs of older people may be less elastic. This can make breathing less efficient, thus reducing oxygen intake. Because the lungs are less efficient, the ribs and the diaphragm do not move as much. This can put older people at risk of chest infections. Other common respiratory problems include (Byrnes 2011: 76):

- Chronic obstructive pulmonary disease (COPD): Over 400,000 people in Ireland are estimated to have this disease
- Cough
- Dyspnoea (breathlessness)
- Influenza (flu): Vaccination is recommended for everyone over 65
- Asthma: Over 477,000 people in Ireland are estimated to have this condition
- Emphysema: Results from a combination of chronic bronchitis and old age
- Lung cancer: Ireland has over twice the EU average of this disease.

The digestive system

As we get older, taste buds and sense of smell become less acute. This may explain why older people have a smaller appetite. Gums recede as we get older, teeth may fall out and there may be less saliva produced in the mouth. A combination of these problems may make eating difficult. The muscles of the digestive system are less effective and food takes longer to pass through, often causing constipation. Nutrients are not absorbed effectively because blood flow is reduced and because some enzymes needed to break down and absorb the nutrients are not produced.

Common problems in the digestive system include:

- Bowel cancer
- Constipation
- Diarrhoea, causing loose stools and pain
- Diverticular disease: Small bubbles in the intestinal lining can pop through the muscular intestinal wall; these are called diverticula and can become inflamed when faecal matter collects in them
- Dysphagia: Difficulties with swallowing, often caused by stroke or neurological disorders
- Haemorrhoids
- Indigestion: This is caused by a range of problems that can occur anywhere along the digestive tract
- Inflammatory bowel disease.

Neurological disorders

Neurological disorders include:

* Dementia
* Motor neurone disease (also known as Lou Gehrig's disease)
* Multiple sclerosis (there are over 7,000 people in Ireland with this condition)
* Parkinson's disease.

Sensory difficulties

Ears

The ear is associated with balance, which may deteriorate due to age, leading to an increase in unsteadiness and falls. Deafness is a common change brought about by ageing. However, deafness can also occur due to disorders or illness. High-frequency tones are often the sounds that are missed by older people.

Conditions that affect the ears include:

* Otitis externa
* Otitis media (middle ear infection)
* Hearing loss.

Sight

Deterioration in eyesight is another common change. As we get older our eyes take longer to react to light and darkness and to change from looking at a distance to looking close up. Cataracts, which cover the lens, may develop, making vision more difficult. Older people find it harder to discriminate between colours, particularly between blue and green.

Conditions that affect the eyes include:

* Cataracts: These form on the lens, making it opaque and affecting vision.
* Glaucoma: This can cause a loss of peripheral vision. It is caused by pressure building up inside the eye.

The four most common health problems experienced by older people today are:

- Heart disease, such as heart attacks and strokes
- Cancer
- Arthritis and other bone diseases
- Brain disease leading to a loss of mental ability.

DEMENTIA

Dementia is a group of related symptoms associated with an ongoing decline of the brain and its ability to function. It affects people's thinking, language, memory, understanding and judgement. According to WHO, the number of people suffering from dementia will triple in the next 40 years, leading to catastrophic social and financial costs. Dementia is a brain illness that affects memory, behaviour and the ability to perform even common tasks, affecting mostly older people. Currently over 5 million people in the US are suffering from dementia (this correlates with vast numbers of people over the age of 80 living in the US). Medical intervention means we are living longer, and the risk of developing dementia increases by 25% after the age of 85 (Byrnes 2011: 47).

The Dementia Services Information and Development Centre states that in Ireland, it is estimated that some 38,000 people are likely to have dementia due to our ageing population. These figures are likely to reach between 80,000 and 100,000 over the next 30 years. Within the HIQA standards there are a set of sub-standards that are dementia specific and require that all services working with people who have a dementia diagnosis will have care plans in place that emphasise autonomy, independence and activity to promote quality of life and well-being.

Listed below are some of the different types of dementia.

- **Alzheimer's disease**, where small clumps of protein, known as plaques, begin to develop around brain cells. This disrupts the normal workings of the brain.
- **Vascular dementia**, where problems with blood circulation result in parts of the brain not receiving enough blood and oxygen.
- **Dementia with Lewy bodies**, where abnormal structures, known as Lewy bodies, develop inside the brain.

♦ **Fronto-temporal dementia**, where the frontal and temporal lobes (two parts of the brain) begin to shrink. Unlike other types of dementia, fronto-temporal dementia usually develops in people who are under 65. It is much rarer than other types of dementia.

Figure 2.2: Symptoms of dementia

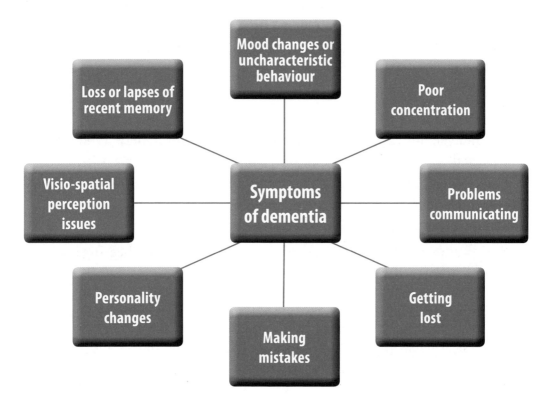

Source: Skills for Care and Skills for Health (2011).

In later stages, these signs will be more pronounced and it can become more difficult for people to live well with dementia.

Common problems for people with dementia include:

♦ Not recognising foods
♦ Forgetting what food they like
♦ Refusing or spitting out food
♦ Resisting being fed
♦ Asking for strange food combinations.

As the number of people with dementia increases, it will be essential that society can enter their world. Person-centred planning is essential in working with people who have dementia. People with this disorder are best understood in the context of their own life history. 'As their dementia progresses, people may be less able to enter our world – we may need to enter theirs and enjoy it with them' (Barbara Pointon, CCA).

According to Gitlin and Corcoran (2005), key person-based contributors to behaviours in the rehabilitation context may include:

* Pain that the individual is unable to identify, understand or articulate as occurring
* Fatigue, poor sleeping patterns
* Fear, anxiety or a sense of a loss of control
* Misunderstandings of the therapeutic process and anxiety as to what is expected
* Underlying incipient medical conditions, such as an infection (e.g. urinary tract infection)
* Clinical depression or psychotic symptoms (hallucinations)
* Significant sensory changes (e.g. reduced visual efficiency, hearing loss)
* Constipation or dehydration.

Key environmental-based factors contributing to behaviours may include:

* A physical environment such as the home or clinic that is too cluttered, distracting and difficult to navigate
* A physical environment that is unfamiliar or too complex, such that the person has difficulty interpreting the meaning of environmental cues and thus responding appropriately
* Presence of others during therapeutic sessions, which may be distracting, confusing and a sensory overload
* Communication patterns that are too complex and confusing.

Dementia and people with a learning disability

Studies carried out by Cooper (1997), as cited in Kerr (2007: 28), show that there has not been much research into the prevalence and incidence of dementia amongst people who have a learning disability. Research that is available suggests that for people with a learning disability with causes other than Down syndrome, there is a prevalence rate higher than would be found in the general population. Studies cited in Kerr (2007: 30) have shown that people with Down syndrome have a much higher rate of Alzheimer's-type dementia than the general population. However, not everyone with Down syndrome will develop the condition. From manifestation to end, this disease could last between eight and 15 years.

As disability services increasingly care for an older population of people due to medical advances, it will be essential that levels of monitoring are higher in these groups.

According to the Alzheimer's Society (2000), as cited by Mathieson (2004), dementia tends to present in people with a learning disability in a similar way to the general population, but early signs are more likely to be missed. Research has also shown that plaques found in brain tissue in certain kinds of dementia contain an amaloid protein that is linked to a gene on chromosome 21, which is significant in the cause of Down syndrome. They state that the incidence is higher in people with a learning disability and suggest that 13% of people aged 50 and over and 22% aged 65 and over are affected – this is around four times the general incidence.

A report, *Home for Good* by Wilkinson et al (2004), paints a bleak picture. Key findings suggest that:

+ A lack of planning leads to unsatisfactory ad hoc arrangements for people with dementia
+ People with dementia had been inappropriately moved to nursing homes due to the lack of coherent strategies to care for them
+ A lack of consistent practice in diagnosis and assessment was evident
+ Good training is crucial and training opportunities varied markedly
+ Staff in all settings struggled with pain management and helping people with dementia to eat.

Communicating with a person with dementia

According to Gitlin et al (2003), the following strategies are recommended:

+ Move and speak slowly and calmly
+ Provide simple one- or two-step verbal instructions at a time
+ Do not rush
+ Allow the patient sufficient time to respond to a command

+ Reassure the person that they are doing a good job
+ Avoid using negative words and negative approaches (don't scold or argue)
+ Eliminate noise and distraction while communicating
+ Be aware of facial expressions; make eye contact but do not stare
+ Express affection – smile, hold hands, give a hug.

IMPACT OF PHYSICAL CHANGES ON EMOTIONAL DEVELOPMENT

As has been previously suggested, sometimes the emotional development of older people is affected by the physical changes that accompany the ageing process. According to Ewles and Simnett, as cited in Schriven and Ewles (2010: 7), there are six dimensions of health: physical, mental, emotional, social, spiritual and societal. This is known as the holistic view of health. Seedhouse (2001), as cited in Schriven and Ewles (2010: 8), proposes an idea of health as the foundation for achieving a person's realistic potential, enabling people to fulfil their own potential. These views demonstrate clearly that health is about empowering individuals to claim responsibility for their own health. We know that this will vary considerably in society. We also know that where individuals are active and responsible agents for their own health, longevity and quality of life are substantially better.

IMPACT OF ILLNESS ON EMOTIONAL DEVELOPMENT

Sometimes the emotional development of older people is affected by illness, either physical or mental. It is sometimes the case that older people feel socially disempowered. The disempowerment of older people can occur by exchange; CCAs may inadvertently enable disempowerment and disablement. It is important when working with the older person to think about what they *can* do. It is important to enable the person to contribute in every possible way, allowing the person to live each day with maximum participation.

It is hard to feel happy and fulfilled when struggling with less mobility, failing eyesight or loss of appetite. Changes in sleep patterns can quickly affect the emotional development of older people and short-term memory loss can be very frustrating. This stage of life may lead to loss of status, a perceived reduced role in life and less contact with friends and colleagues from work.

Other factors that may impact on the mental health of this age group include a gradual deterioration in health and physical capability, loss of financial stability, changing environments (moving home) and a loss of the sense of 'belonging' and other social and psychological factors.

It is not all negative, however. For some, advancing years can mean a time of freedom from the grind of employment, the child-rearing years and other responsibilities. It can offer an opportunity to do the things they hadn't had time to do before and a chance to develop new social contacts. In some cultures, reaching old age might mean increased social status.

Task

Imagine for a moment that you had to leave your own home and go into a nursing home. How would you feel? What would you bring with you?

CCAs AND OLDER PEOPLE

The qualities of a CCA will include:

- Being a good listener
- Being able to put yourself in someone else's shoes (empathy)
- Knowing how to treat people as individuals
- Keeping a confidence (if appropriate) and being aware of the feelings of others.

Good CCAs can observe the needs of their client and show patience, allowing the individual time and assisting the person to maintain independence, and will be capable of treating people with respect.

There are a number of important interpersonal skills that will help the CCA understand and support the needs of the older person. Interpersonal skills are behaviours that help and encourage people to communicate, to understand, to be understood and to express their needs, thoughts and feelings. As we get older we tend to become more dependent on other people, so it is therefore very important that CCAs do all they can to ensure the needs of the older person are met. This book places a great emphasis on therapeutic communication. It is the cornerstone of good care.

Confidentiality

It is essential for the older person to trust people, especially their CCA. It is therefore very important that confidentiality is maintained. Everyone has the right to privacy. Information given to you should only be passed on if the individual gives you permission to do so. If the confidence involves something legal or may cause harm to someone, the information may need to be shared – always take advice from a supervisor or senior member of staff. Refer to Chapter 6 for further information.

Task

Have you ever told a friend something in confidence, only to find out later that they told someone else? How did you feel? Would you confide in them again?

Communicating with older people

It is important that our personal communication styles and behaviour are incorporated into our self-reflection in order to enhance our overall clinical performance. According to Berglund and Saltman (2002), we all need to recognise our own preferred way of communicating in order to determine our own strengths and weaknesses. We need to look at ourselves first before we can become effective communicators with others. You will need to note that your communication style will differ according to the audience (for example, family interactions will differ from interactions at work).

Always ensure that you compliment and acknowledge the person. It is imperative that you develop a relationship that provides comfort, is honest and conveys a positive attitude. It is essential to explain, providing a clear rationale for every procedure, ensuring at all times that privacy, confidentiality and feelings of independence are respected. For more detailed understanding of the importance of communicating appropriately with an older person, refer to Chapter 6.

SAFEGUARDING OLDER PEOPLE

According to the HSE (2002), elder abuse is defined as 'a single or repeated act, or lack of appropriate action, occurring within any relationship where there is an expectation of trust which causes harm or distress to an older person or violates their human and civil rights'.

A study carried out by Naughton et al (2012) over a 12-month period examined the prevalence of elder abuse and neglect in community-dwelling older people in Ireland and examined the risk profile of people who experienced mistreatment and that of the perpetrators. This study showed that the prevalence of elder abuse and neglect was 2.2%. The types of mistreatment were financial (1.3%), psychological (1.2%), physical abuse (0.5%), neglect (0.3%) and sexual abuse (0.05%). It is worth noting that neglect is often unrecognised and sexual abuse is not reported.

Older people are more vulnerable and consequently are susceptible to abuse. It is important that CCAs can identify signs, risk factors and possible causes of abuse. There are four types of abuse: physical, psychological/emotional, sexual and financial. Abuse can occur in the person's own home or in an institutional setting, such as a residential home, day service or hospital. Perpetrators can be a partner, relative, friend, CCA or volunteer.

Physical abuse

Physical abuse is physical force or violence that results in bodily injury, pain or impairment. It includes assault, battery and inappropriate restraint. Physical abuse includes:

- Grabbing, shaking, pushing, pinching, hair pulling, hitting, etc.
- Withholding food or drink
- Inappropriate supervision
- Restraining inappropriately
- Failure to provide aids, glasses, dentures and frames.

Signs of physical abuse: Bruises, burns, lacerations, hypothermia, dehydration, malnutrition, poor hygiene, weight loss, inexplicable falls, old wounds.

Psychological/emotional abuse

Psychological/emotional abuse is like brainwashing in that it systematically wears away at the victim's self-confidence, sense of self-worth, trust in their own perceptions and self-concept. Whether it is done by constant berating and belittling, by intimidation or under the guise of 'guidance', 'teaching' or 'advice', the results are similar. Psychological/emotional abuse includes:

+ Verbal abuse, shouting, teasing, swearing, name calling
+ Ignoring the person
+ Causing the person to feel ashamed (especially commenting on bowel movements or incontinence).

Signs of psychological/emotional abuse: Insomnia, loss of appetite, weight loss, loss of self-esteem, confusion.

Sexual abuse

Sexual abuse is any misuse of a child or adult for sexual pleasure or gratification. Sexual abuse includes:

+ Teasing
+ Touching
+ Kissing
+ Caressing
+ Molesting
+ Rape.

Signs of sexual abuse: Bruising, pain, anal or vaginal bleeding, difficulty walking or sitting, overt sexuality, especially in confused people, sexually transmitted diseases.

Task

Read the HSE document *Open Your Eyes*. Think about what is expected of you if you witness abuse.

Financial abuse

Financial abuse is the improper taking or misuse of the money or property of a vulnerable adult for the benefit of someone other than the vulnerable adult. The term 'financial abuse' describes the situation where an abuser:

* Is borrowing money from a vulnerable adult
* Is refusing to give a vulnerable adult access to his/her money.

Signs of financial abuse: Personal belongings go missing, disparity between income and living conditions.

Neglect

The HSE defines neglect as a 'type of maltreatment that refers to the failure to provide needed age-appropriate care', such as shelter, food, clothing, education, supervision, medical care and other basic necessities needed for the development of physical, intellectual and emotional capacities. Signs of neglect include:

* Malnutrition due to insufficient monitoring of nutritional needs
* Physical harm in the form of cuts, bruises and burns due to lack of supervision
* Passive restraint, bed bound, chair bound or left alone for long periods of time.

Medical neglect is the failure to provide appropriate health care for a person when financially able to do so. Medical neglect can result in poor overall health and compounded medical problems.

Living with neglect can significantly increase the person's chances of becoming ill or dying early. The stress of living with abuse or neglect may also make other health problems worse.

Many vulnerable adults who experience neglect also face emotional and/ or financial abuse. This can lead to ongoing distress in the person's life. If the abuser controls the vulnerable person's money, they may have fewer resources to take care of their own health, secure and maintain proper housing or obtain good nutrition and participate in healthy activities.

Task

Consider your own thoughts and feelings about abuse of older adults.

How do we prevent abuse?

The most successful way of preventing abuse in older people is to make them aware of what constitutes abuse. Very often the perpetrators of abuse are family and it is difficult for the victim to actually accept that the person will behave in this way.

+ Take all reports of abuse seriously.
+ Treat all those involved with respect.
+ Respect confidentiality.
+ Always seek consent before taking any action.
+ Remember, the victim is an adult and is free to decide. People may choose to continue in a situation that is abusive.

The appropriate action to take is to contact the GP, public health nurse or senior case worker or phone the HSE information line on 1850 241 850.

DEATH AND DYING

In the 21st century, dying is a changing experience. Degenerative long-term diseases now mean that we need to change our approach and think about the experience of dying. Diagnosis of diseases that lead to cognitive impairment means we need to allow people to think about this process much earlier.

According to *DML Services for Older People*:

Chronic diseases and terminal diseases are the common reason for adopting a palliative care approach. People with life-limiting, non-malignant diseases can experience a range of physical and psychological symptoms throughout the course of their disease. Their symptom burden has been shown to be equal to that of people dying with cancer. In addition, their disease process can be more complex and often of a much longer duration. These aspects of non-malignant disease demonstrate the need for a palliative care approach to be incorporated as part of their routine care.

Some life-limiting diseases that require particular consideration for palliative care include:

* Dementia
* Heart failure
* Advanced respiratory disease, such as COPD
* Chronic kidney disease
* Motor neurone disease
* Cardiovascular accident
* Multiple sclerosis.

It will be important to assess symptoms. Areas of concern will include:

* Pain management
* Communication
* Equipment
* Wishes
* Dignity, respect and privacy
* Decision-making ability, for example, around resuscitation
* Information
* Support services that may be required by family
* Conflict management of current or potential issues
* Cultural beliefs and practices
* Legal implications of life being withheld or withdrawn
* Spiritual beliefs and wishes.

BEREAVEMENT

It is essential when working with older people that we can guard against depression, so we need to observe and support individuals who experience the loss of a significant other. It can be the case that following the loss of a significant other after a chronic and protracted illness, the spouse may have been so immersed and absorbed by the needs of the other person that they have entirely neglected their own needs. It is important to support people and direct people towards support groups and bereavement counselling as necessary.

Another consideration for older people is the level of bereavement faced by many older people. They may lose family or friends and this is sometimes sudden, such as an accident or heart attack, or after a long illness such as cancer. Grieving is a difficult process and older people need help and understanding in dealing with their emotions.

DEPRESSION

Ageing brings with it enormous developmental challenges. The loss of significant others, loss of function and reduction in independence can all lead to depression. It is essential that the mental health of older people is promoted through activation programmes that will enhance and support their social and emotional health. Older people have traditionally gained support through spiritual groups, which enhance social contact for people generally. Increasingly in Irish society, attachment to spiritual groups may be in decline, and this support network, which has played a significant role in the socialisation of older people, needs consideration. Depression and its signs and symptoms will be dealt with in greater detail in Chapter 5.

When we are communicating with older people who are grieving, it is important to employ an empathetic approach to get a sense of their feelings and emotions. We must listen and allow the person to speak, but also allow the person to be silent.

SUMMARY

This chapter illustrates how important our perceptions of ageing are when working with older people. Examination of the ageing process helps us to understand the dimensions of health and their interactions in the maintenance or deterioration of health. It is essential that all those working with older people understand diseases such as dementia and can recognise problems that arise in the safeguarding of older adults. This chapter concludes with an identification of some of the issues faced by older adults at the end of life.

REFERENCES

Berglund, C.A. and Saltman, D. (eds) (2002) *Communication for Health Care*, Melbourne: Oxford University Press.

Byrnes, N. (2011) *Your Health Matters*, Dublin: Blackwater Press.

Department of Health and Children (2009) Health Act 2007 (Care and Welfare of Residents in Designated Centres for Older People) Regulations 2009, Dublin: Stationery Office.

Department of Health and Children (2010) Health Act 2007 (Care and Welfare of Residents in Designated Centres for Older People) (Amendment) Regulations 2010, Dublin: Stationery Office.

Gitlin, L. and Corcoran, M. (2005) *Occupational Therapy and Dementia Care: The Home Environmental Skill-building Program for Individuals and Families*, Bethesda, MD: American Occupational Therapy Association.

Gitlin, L., Liebman, J. and Winter, L. (2003) 'Are environmental interventions effective in the management of Alzheimer's disease and related disorders? A synthesis of the evidence', *Alzheimer's Care Quarterly*, 4(2), pp. 85–107.

HIQA (2009) *National Quality Standards for Residential Care Settings for Older People in Ireland*, HIQA.

HSE (2002) *Protecting Our Future: Report of the Working Group on Elder Abuse*, Dublin: Stationery Office.

HSE (2011) 'What is elder abuse?', available online at www.hse.ie (accessed 8 November 2012).

Kerr, D. (2007) *Understanding Learning Disability and Dementia*, London: Athenaeum Press, pp. 14–21.

Mathieson, A. (2004) 'Learning disability and dementia', *Learning Disability Practice*, 7(7), pp. 12–13.

National Council for Ageing and Older People (NCAOP) (2004) *Population in Ireland: Projections 2002–2021*. Dublin: NCAOP.

Naughton, C. et al (2012) 'Elder abuse and neglect in Ireland: Results from a national prevalence survey', *Age and Ageing*, 41(1), pp. 98–103.

NHS (2009) *Common Core Principles to Support Self Care: A Guide to Support Implementation*, Leeds: Skills for Care. www.skillsforcare.org.uk

Schriven, A. (2010) *Promoting Health: A Practical Guide*, 6th edition, Oxford: Bailliere Tindall/Elsevier, pp. 6–8.

Schriven, A. and Ewles, L. (2010) *Promoting Health: A Practical Guide*, 6th edition, Edinburgh: Bailliere Tindall/Elsevier.

Skills for Care and Skills for Health (2011) *Common Core Principles for Supporting People with Dementia*, Leeds (www.skillsforcare.org.uk, www.skillsforhealth.org.uk).

Strydom, A., Hassiotis, A., King, M. and Livingston, G. (2009) 'The relationship of dementia prevalence in older adults with intellectual disability (ID) to age and severity of ID', *Psychological Medicine*, 39, pp. 13–21.

Tyas, S.L., Snowdon, D.A., Desrosiers, M.F., Riley, K.P. and Markesbery, W.R. (2007) 'Healthy ageing in the nun study: Definition and neuropathologic correlates', *Age and Ageing*, 36(6), pp. 650–5.

Wilkinson, H., Kerr, D., Cunningham, C. and Rae, C. (2004) *Home for Good? Models of Good Practice for Supporting People with a Learning Disability and Dementia*, Brighton: Pavilion Press.

Zaretsky, H., Richter, E. and Eisenberg, M. (2005) *Medical Aspects of Disability: A Handbook for the Rehabilitation Profession*, 3rd edition, New York: Springer Publishing, pp. 292–3.

3
Disability Awareness

INTRODUCTION

This chapter explores the concept of disability by defining it and breaking it down to examine the various types of disability and how living with a disability affects people's day-to-day experience. This chapter will provide you with the knowledge needed to provide individualised person-centred care. As professionals working in the health care setting, we care for many different people. It is important to remember that every person we meet is unique and therefore the care they receive should be tailored to their specific needs.

KEY TERMS

- acquired brain injury
- assistive aids
- autism
- cerebral palsy
- challenging behaviour
- diabetes
- Down syndrome
- epilepsy
- pervasive developmental disorder
- sensory loss

WHAT IS DISABILITY?

The World Health Organisation (WHO) offers the following description of disability:

Disability is an umbrella term, covering impairments, activity limitations, and participation restrictions. An impairment is a problem in body function or structure; an activity limitation is a difficulty encountered by an individual in executing a task or action; while a participation restriction is a problem experienced by an individual in involvement in life situations. Thus disability is a complex phenomenon, reflecting an interaction between features of a person's body and features of the society in which he or she lives.

At one point or another in our lives, we will have or will experience an impairment, be it temporary or permanent. It will be helpful to keep that experience in mind while studying this chapter.

THE HISTORY OF DISABILITY IN IRELAND

For most of this century the closed doors of institutions, sheltered workshops and long stay hospitals concealed disability from public view. (Silvers et al 1998)

The traditional focus on people with disabilities has been on their deficits and addressing those deficits through the provision of group-based services. This segregated people with disabilities from the general community (HSE 2011). This type of service provision reinforces social exclusion and does not empower individuals to exercise choice and control over their lives.

The work of voluntary bodies, families of and people with disabilities campaigning for civil rights, equality and inclusion has been the driving force behind societal and attitude changes. Ireland has progressed and people with disabilities are more integrated into Irish society. The recent results of the 2012 Paralympics are testament to these improvements.

In 2003, the European Year of People with Disabilities put the spotlight on Ireland's antiquated disability services and highlighted the lack of legislation that would uphold the rights of people with disabilities (Hyde, Lohan and McDonnell 2004).

The social model of disability

Sometimes people with disabilities are often prevented from full participation in the community and from achieving their full potential by the attitudes of others or the barriers created by society. These barriers can restrict access to important facilities, such as public transport, entertainment and public places, education or employment. The focus needs to change – the onus is on Irish society to eliminate barriers and make it possible for everyone to participate fully.

Integrated services

People with disabilities are entitled to access the same public services as non-disabled people. The law says that public services for people with disabilities should be integrated with services for other people where it is practical and appropriate. Benefits of providing integrated services for everybody include increased presence and participation within the community, which leads to further acceptance and integration. Further, more people with disabilities can be empowered by the positive and meaningful contributions they can make to their community. Finally, it is only through community integration that the stigma and discrimination associated with disability will be addressed.

LEGISLATION

The Disability Act 2005 is a key element of Ireland's National Disability Strategy. Among other measures, this Act requires public bodies to make their buildings, information and services accessible for people with disabilities.

Providers of goods and services (including education and housing) must accommodate the needs of people with disabilities by making reasonable changes in what they do and how they do it.

These Acts prohibit discrimination in recruitment, employment and training on nine grounds, including disability. Employers are legally obliged to provide employees with disabilities with reasonable accommodation to enable them to do their job, unless the cost would be disproportionate.

This Act provides for children with special education needs to attend a mainstream school with other students, unless this is not consistent with the best interest of the child or the effective provision of educational services for other children.

Part 3 of the Disability Act 2005 provides that by law, public bodies must:

♦ Ensure that people with disabilities can use their services easily and at the same location or access point as everyone else.

- Provide information in a way that suits the needs of people with disabilities, for example by phone, by email, in plain English, large print or in Braille. Websites must also meet specified accessibility standards.
- Ensure, where possible, that goods and services they buy or hire can be used by people with disabilities.
- Have accessible premises by 2015.

Additionally, part 3 of the Act included sectoral plans for six government departments:

- Communications, Energy and Natural Resources
- Enterprise, Trade and Employment
- Environment and Local Government
- Health
- Social and Family Affairs
- Transport.

Unfortunately, due to the economic downturn, many services for people with disabilities have been targeted for savings and advocacy groups continue to protest for services to be maintained and targets to be met.

PREVALENCE AND TYPES OF DISABILITY

The National Disability Survey 2006 presents a detailed analysis of the numbers of people affected by disability and the prevalence of each disability. Most disability is acquired through the life course rather than being present from birth or childhood. An intellectual and learning disability is the exception in that it peaks in the early teens. This form of disability is more likely to be noted during the school years and is more frequently diagnosed now than in the past (Watson and Nolan 2011).

The survey distinguishes nine different types of disability. The average person with a disability may have a mix of these different types of disabilities or a dual diagnosis.

1. Mobility and dexterity disability, which includes difficulties in walking, lifting and carrying things and in picking up small objects (about 184,000 people)

2. Pain (about 153,000 people)

3. Remembering and concentrating disability (113,000 people)

4. Emotional, psychological and mental health disabilities (111,000)

5. Intellectual and learning disability (72,000)

6. Breathing disability (71,000)

7. Hearing disability (58,000)

8. Vision disability (51,000)

9. Speech disabilities (35,000) (Watson and Nolan 2011)

This survey aids services in the planning and distribution of funding to areas of need. The survey classifies disability under the nine terms above, but in this chapter we will examine the concept of disability under the following headings.

Figure 3.1: Chapter overview

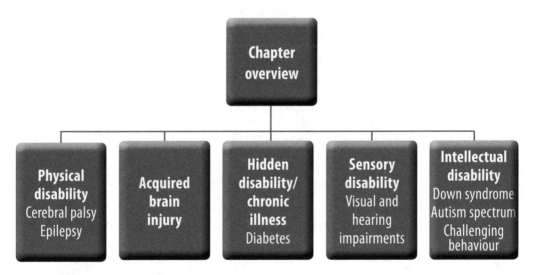

PHYSICAL DISABILITY

Physical disability pertains to total or partial loss of a person's bodily function or total or partial loss of a part of the body (e.g. a person with an amputation).

Examples of physical disability include:

+ Amputation
+ Cerebral palsy

+ Multiple sclerosis
+ Muscular dystrophy
+ Acquired spinal injury (paraplegia or quadriplegia).

People with a disability are able to lead rich and fulfilling lives – their main obstacles are the ones created by society. People with physical disabilities have normal comprehension and intelligence, but they often report being treated as though they have impaired intelligence. People with disabilities report being ignored in a three-way conversation and having their own views overlooked. People like Joanne O'Riordan, who at the young age of 15 challenged Taoiseach Enda Kenny regarding budget cuts to disability funding, have had a tremendous impact on this perception and are leading the way forward. Equally, the London 2012 Olympics gave more emphasis to the Paralympics than any other Olympic event in history, which is evidence that this perception is changing.

The societal mindset of pity for people with disabilities is not inclusive. People with physical disabilities have the same priorities as anyone else, e.g. career, rent, mortgage, family, socialising.

Sometimes the way our communities are set up create barriers for people with disabilities to lead full and productive lives. For example, in Ireland some major cities have made great improvements in regards to upgrading transport facilities, but many towns and rural areas remain inaccessible for people with physical disabilities (Watson and Nolan 2011).

Epilepsy

Epilepsy is defined as a disorder of the brain characterised by an ongoing liability to recurrent epileptic seizures (Shorvon 2009).

The brain is made of millions of nerve cells, or neurons. Their activity is organised and rhythmic. The brain is responsible for a wide range of functions, such as movement, consciousness, storing and recalling memory. It is usually well organised and possesses mechanisms for self-regulation.

What is a seizure?

A seizure is a brief excessive discharge of brain electrical activity that changes how a person feels, senses, thinks or behaves (Devinsky 2007).

A seizure is often called a fit, an attack, a turn or a blackout. Electrical activity is present within the brain all the time. A seizure occurs when there is a sudden burst of excess electrical activity (Bingham 2011). Seizures can take many forms. The way in which a seizure manifests depends on its origin within the brain and how far it spreads.

Generalised seizures

There are six categories of generalised seizures. In each of them, consciousness is impaired and motor changes on both sides, or hemispheres, of the brain are affected (Appleton and Marson 2009).

Partial seizures

These are seizures that arise in one specific part of the brain. One hemisphere, or side, of the brain is affected. There are two types of partial seizures: simple and complex (Shorvon 2009).

Table 3.1: Types of seizures

Generalised seizures	Partial seizures
Absence	Simple partial
Myoclonic jerking	Complex partial
Clonic	
Tonic	
Tonic-clonic	
Atonic	

Status epilepticus (SE)

This is a life-threatening condition. Good first aid is essential to prevent severe brain damage or mortality. It is a condition in which epileptic seizures continue or repeat without recovery for a period of 30 minutes or more (Shorvon 2009). Treatment is generally started after the seizure has lasted five minutes. This varies from person to person. Each person with epilepsy is unique and should have an individualised care plan regarding their care during a seizure from their GP or neurologist as to how long a carer or family member should wait before giving rescue medication. Training in the appropriate administration of such medication is essential and should be assessed before a person is deemed competent to administer either of the medications listed below, as it is always considered a medicalemergency.

There are two commonly used forms of rescue medication:

+ **Diazepam**, also known as Stesolid, which is administered rectally
+ **Buccal Midazolam**, also known as Epistatus, which is administered into the buccal mucosa.

If a person has a history of SE, they should carry their rescue medication with them everywhere, provided they are accompanied by a person who has been trained in its administration.

There is a risk of death or severe brain damage while a person is in SE, especially if treatment is not initiated quickly enough.

Aura

Some people with epilepsy experience what's known as an aura before a seizure. It can occur at any time leading up to the seizure. An aura is individual to each person and not every person with epilepsy experiences an aura. However, for the person who does experience it, it often gives them time to lie down in a safe place to prevent themselves from falling and injuring themselves during the seizure.

Some people experience the following:

+ Vision, smell or sounds
+ Anxiety/fear
+ Nausea
+ Weakness
+ Tingling of a limb or limbs.

Diagnosis

Epilepsy is diagnosed on a good history taken from someone who has witnessed a seizure. Investigations such as EEG (electroencephalography) help with classification but cannot substitute for good history-taking.

All anti-epileptic drugs cross the blood–brain barrier. All therefore have the potential to produce adverse effects on alertness, cognition and mental state.

Finally, epilepsy can have a considerable social impact, potentially leading to overprotection, stigmatisation and secondary handicap and low self-esteem.

Treatment

All epilepsy treatment is a balance between risk and benefit (Shorvon 2010). The aim of treatment is for the patient to be seizure free, preferably on a single anti-epileptic drug (AED), and to be free of adverse drug side effects. The effect of the AED is generally assessed by measuring its impact on seizure frequency (Shorvon 2010).

Having epilepsy involves far more than the risk of recurrent seizures. It incorporates prejudice, stigmatisation, psychological and social issues that may be more problematic than the seizures themselves (Shorvon 2010). It is also important to note the psychological impact of living with epilepsy. The sudden loss of independence and fear of leaving one's home alone may be shrouded in anxieties and can lead to social isolation.

Cerebral palsy

Cerebral palsy (CP) is a commonly used term for a group of conditions characterised by motor dysfunction due to non-progressive brain damage early in life (Levitt 2010). Cerebral palsy is a lifelong condition that can range from mild to severe in degree (Bjorklund 2007). It is classified under the following headings: athetoid or dyskinetic, ataxic and spastic.

Figure 3.2: Cerebral palsy

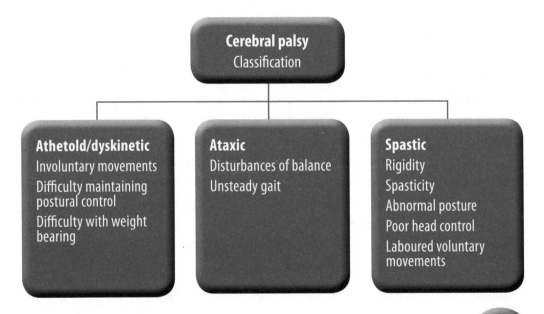

The terms 'spastic' or 'spasticity' are generally used by clinicians to describe muscle stiffness (Levitt 2010).

Causes

CP occurs as a result of damage to the parts of the brain that control movement. The damage that causes CP is thought to occur either before or during birth:

+ Lack of oxygen at birth (anoxia)
+ Infection
+ Premature birth
+ Cerebral bleeds
+ Trauma or accident at a young age while the brain is still developing.

Treatment and management of symptoms

When planning the care and management of individuals with cerebral palsy, the goal is not to cure or to achieve normalcy, but to increase functionality, improve capabilities and sustain health in terms of locomotion, cognitive development, social interaction and independence (Krigger 2006). Physical symptoms of CP are treated through physiotherapy, occupational therapy and often hydrotherapy. Depending on the level of muscle stiffness or rigidity, treatment may consist of oral muscle relaxant medication (e.g. Baclofen) and injections of Botox into affected muscles. Assistive aids and technological advances enable and empower people with CP to lead fuller, more independent lives.

ACQUIRED BRAIN INJURY (ABI)

The brain has been described as a machine, a matrix, a jungle or a desktop computer, while the mind is noted as a container, a multipurpose tool or the self (Fernyhough 2005). ABI can result in cognitive, physical, emotional or behavioural impairments that lead to permanent or temporary changes in functioning (Woodward and Waterhouse 2009). There are two categories of brain injury: traumatic and non-traumatic. It is important to remember that every brain injury is unique to each person; Table 3.2 is not an exhaustive list.

Figure 3.3: Types and causes of acquired brain injury

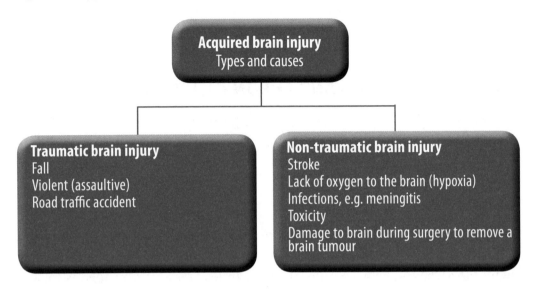

Table 3.2: Conditions associated with ABI

Cognition	Slowed processing and co-ordination of thoughts
Sensory	Confusing or painful effects from 'ordinary' overload but overwhelming sensory stimuli, e.g. sound
Anxiety	Becoming excessively anxious, whether for real or imagined causes
Fatigue	Easily tired (but often unaware of being so), then sharply dropping mental performance
Attention	Easy and agitated distractibility
Memory	Poor or jumbled recall
Sleep	Long-term difficulty in getting restful sleep
Communicating	Difficulty with word-finding and expression

Management

Long-term management presents a unique challenge to a multidisciplinary team. Management must be person centred, taking into consideration the individual's preferences and maintaining their dignity, self-respect and decision-making abilities (Woodward and Waterhouse 2009), and guided by the individual's needs and goals.

Rehabilitation following an acquired brain injury does not follow a set protocol due to the complexity and variable nature of each injury.

Care must be provided on an individual basis. No two patients will present with the same motor, cognitive, physiological or psychological response to the injury (Woodward and Waterhouse 2009).

HIDDEN DISABILITIES AND CHRONIC ILLNESS

Mental illness is the most common hidden disability in Irish society (see Chapter 5 for more on this topic). The second most common hidden disability is diabetes.

Diabetes

Diabetes is a medical condition where there is too much sugar or glucose circulating in the bloodstream. The body regulates glucose levels precisely; high glucose levels over a period of time can lead to health problems for the individual. The hormone that controls glucose levels is insulin. Insulin is manufactured in the pancreas. Insulin deficiency is the mechanism behind diabetes (Matthews et al 2008). The pancreas is a gland behind the stomach. When food is digested and enters your bloodstream, insulin moves any glucose out of the blood and into cells, where it is broken down to produce energy. People with diabetes are unable to break down glucose into energy. This is because there is either not enough insulin to move the glucose or because the insulin that is there does not work properly.

There are two types of diabetes: type I and type II.

Table 3.3: Types of diabetes

Type I diabetes	Type II diabetes
Juvenile	Older age
Abrupt onset	Gradual onset
Family history	Family history
Autoimmune (a condition where the body confuses insulin-producing cells for foreign or infected cells and destroys them)	Insulin deficiency
Insulin dependent	

Figure 3.4: Symptoms of diabetes

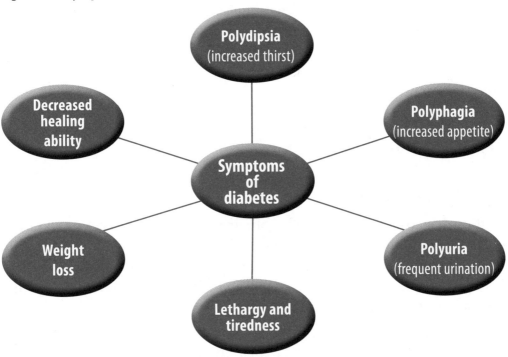

People with diabetes must also make sure that their blood glucose levels stay balanced by eating a healthy diet and carrying out regular blood tests.

Figure 3.5: Diabetes management and care

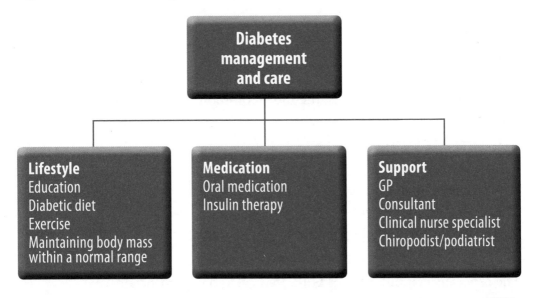

The ill health experienced by individuals with diabetes can have implications for how they function in their community (Holt et al 2011). The physical differences that occur with diabetes may impair one's ability to perform domestic tasks and assume societal roles. As a result, diabetes may inhibit a person's ability to fully integrate into society and thus can be considered a hidden disability.

SENSORY DISABILITY

Visual impairments

Medical diagnostic guidelines define blindness as no light perception (NLP). It refers to a person who is unable to recognise any light. Blindness is frequently used to describe severe visual impairment with residual vision. Those described as having only light perception have the ability to tell light from dark and the general direction of a light source (Sardegna et al 2002).

'Visual impairment' is a term used to describe a person who has sight loss in one or both eyes. Various scales have been developed to describe the extent of visual impairment.

There are four levels of visual function, according to the International Classification of Diseases:

+ Normal vision
+ Moderate visual impairment
+ Severe visual impairment
+ Blindness.

According to WHO estimates, the most common causes of blindness around the world in 2002 were:

+ Cataracts (47.9%)
+ Glaucoma (12.3%)
+ Age-related macular degeneration (8.7%)
+ Corneal opacity (5.1%)
+ Diabetic retinopathy (4.8%).

The experience of blindness is both physical and psychosocial.

Table 3.4: Physical and psychosocial aspects of blindness

Physical aspects	Psychosocial aspects
Cause	Psychological effect of a new diagnosis
Diagnosis	Adjustment
Prognosis	Adapted learning and education
Prescription (corrective lenses)	Adaptation to environment

Figure 3.6: Assistive aids

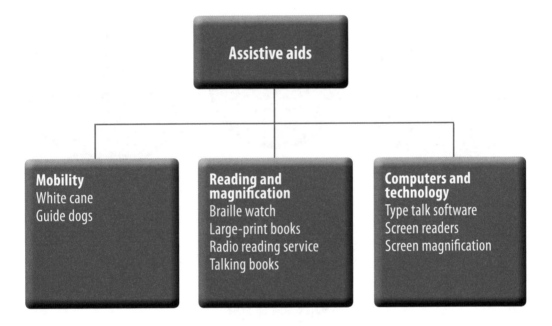

Deafness

Deafness refers to the complete loss of hearing in one or both ears. Hearing impairment refers to both complete and partial loss of the ability to hear (WHO 2011).

There are two types of hearing impairment (WHO 2012):

♦ **Conductive:** Hearing impairment affects outer or middle ear.

♦ **Sensorineural:** Hearing impairment affects inner ear or hearing nerve.

Figure 3.7: Hearing aids assistive technology

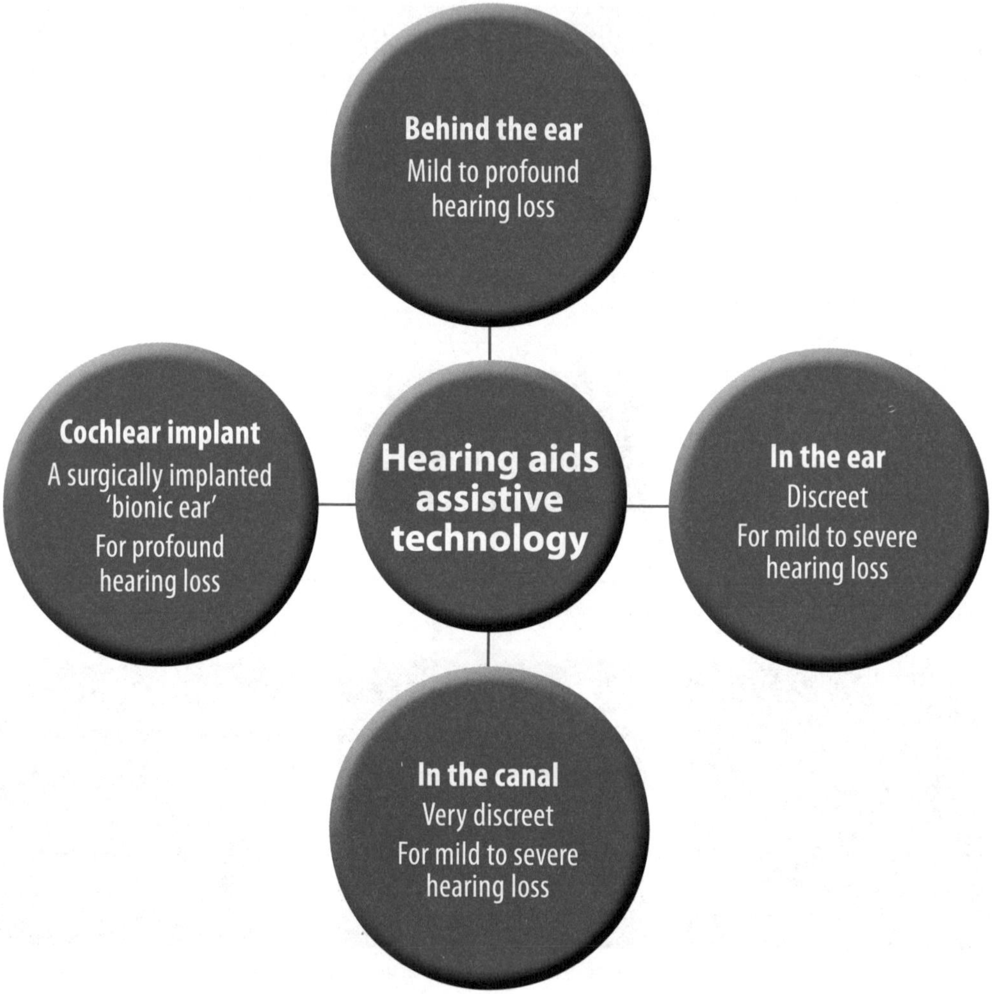

Behind the ear
Mild to profound hearing loss

Cochlear implant
A surgically implanted 'bionic ear'
For profound hearing loss

Hearing aids assistive technology

In the ear
Discreet
For mild to severe hearing loss

In the canal
Very discreet
For mild to severe hearing loss

INTELLECTUAL DISABILITY

Intellectual disability is defined as a substantial limitation in present functioning. It is characterised by significantly sub-average intellectual functioning (IQ < 75) existing in conjunction with related limitations in two or more of the following applicable adaptive skills: communication, self-care, social skills, community use, self-direction, health and safety, functional academics, leisure and work. Intellectual disability manifests itself before the age of 18 (Lukasson et al 1992, cited in Emerson 2001).

Gates (2003) identifies intellectual disability by the presence of a significantly reduced ability to understand new or complex information with a reduced ability to cope independently.

Table 3.5: Classification of intellectual disability

Mild intellectual disability	IQ 50–70
Moderate intellectual disability	IQ 35–55
Severe intellectual disability	IQ 20–40
Profound intellectual disability	IQ 20–25

Source: Adapted from DSM-IVTR, a globally recognised diagnostic tool.

Figure 3.8: Causes of intellectual disability

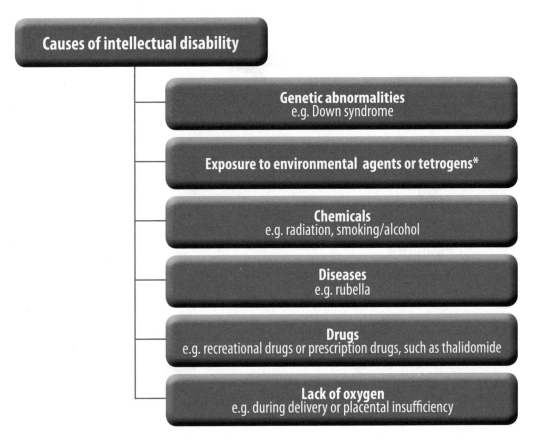

*Tetrogens are agents that cause changes in normal pre-natal development. Foetal development can be damaged by tetrogenic exposure.

Management

The needs of people with intellectual disabilities are always changing. People with intellectual disabilities learn throughout their lives and can continue to obtain skills with the help of their caregivers. Figure 3.9 illustrates five core domains of care management. Each domain is reliant on the others. If one aspect is neglected, all others are affected. If we are to maintain a holistic approach to care, equal time and resources should be given to each domain. Often as a result of short staffing, a greater emphasis is placed on physical care and personal hygiene. While this is essential to health and well-being, in order to be truly holistic and empower the individuals in our care, every aspect of the person should be catered to if they are to reach their fullest potential.

Figure 3.9: Domains of care management in intellectual disability

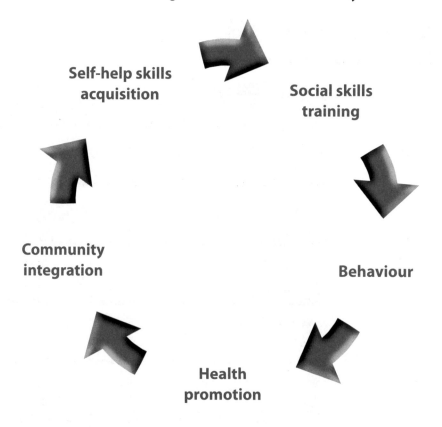

Self-help skills
acquisition

Social skills
training

Community
integration

Behaviour

Health
promotion

Down syndrome

A syndrome is a condition distinguished by a cluster of features occurring together. If a person has a number of the features associated with that particular syndrome, he or she is said to have that syndrome (Selikowitz 2008). Down syndrome (DS) is a chromosomal condition caused by the presence of all or part of a third copy of chromosome 21. It is typically associated with a delay in cognitive ability, intellectual disability (ID) and physical growth and a particular set of facial and physical characteristics. Down syndrome is the most common chromosome abnormality in humans (Jacobsen Bosch 2003). The list in Figure 3.10 is not exhaustive and not all features will be present in each person.

Figure 3.10: Physical features of Down syndrome

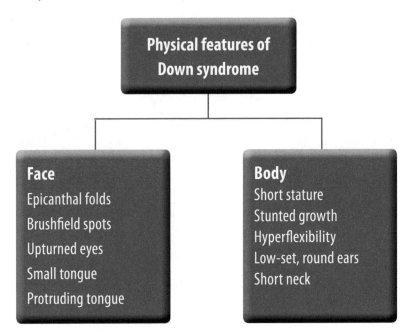

Conditions associated with Down syndrome

Adults with Down syndrome should be offered all the regular screening tests and health care maintenance interventions that are commonly provided to adults who do not have Down syndrome (Urbano 2010). People with Down syndrome may have an unusual presentation of an ordinary illness or condition.

Behaviour changes or loss of function may be the only indication of medical illness (Smith 2001).

Figure 3.11: Conditions associated with Down syndrome

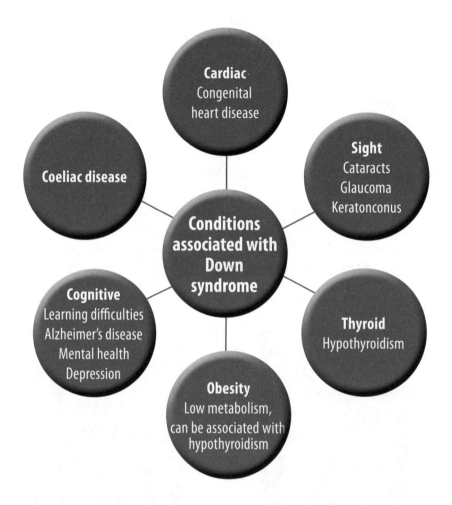

Adolescence

People with DS will experience the rush of hormones in exactly the same way as other teenagers. This can be a difficult time and will need to be carefully negotiated and understood. This includes adolescents trying to establish their own identity and being given opportunities to explore. Attempts to hold the teenager back may result in conflict and behavioural difficulties. It is very important to understand people with DS as having life span development and not to stereotype the individual by holding onto the eternal child label (Selikowitz 2008).

Menarche tends to be related to the timing of menarche in the mother (Jacobsen Bosch 2003). Menstruation usually settles into a regular pattern. Consideration should be given to the possibility of premenstrual syndrome in women with cyclic irritability, aggression or self-harm (Jacobsen Bosch 2003). As in other teenage girls, ovulation still takes place, so fertility should be presumed. Women with DS have borne children, so discussions regarding sexuality and contraception are very important (Van Dyke et al 1997). More enlightened thinking has allowed women with DS to successfully manage their own menses and to make decisions about contraception.

Adolescent boys with DS usually experience the same sexual drives and frustrations as their peers. Masturbation occurs in people with DS, just as in the general population. Efforts should be directed towards privacy rather than trying to stop the behaviour (Van Dyke et al 1997).

Adulthood

Changes in the approach to people with Down syndrome in the latter part of the 20th century has resulted in a threefold increase in their life expectancy, largely due to better and more active medical care coupled with community living (Urbano 2010). This means that medical practitioners need to employ the same preventive health skills as they do for the rest of the community. In addition, a man of 25 should not be called a 'boy'. He has usually moved out of the family home and is working in an adult day service or supported employment. He is probably able to answer questions about his health and should be given the opportunity to do so. He is an adult and should be treated as such (Carr 1995).

Behavioural changes

Behavioural changes are often identified in later life. There are number of situations that may cause such changes:

* Difficulty with transitions in adulthood
* Leaving school, resulting in a loss of social networks
* Departure of older siblings from the family home
* Loss and bereavement
* Moves from home to community or residential settings

+ Development of vision or hearing impairments
+ Hypothyroidism
+ Mental health issues
+ Alzheimer's disease.

Any significant change or life event should be considered when establishing a cause for behaviour change (see the 'Challenging behaviour' section at the end of this chapter). While Alzheimer's disease occurs earlier and more often in adults with Down syndrome than in the general population, not every behavioural or cognitive change in an adult with Down syndrome should be ascribed to this form of dementia.

Care management in adulthood

+ Auditory testing (every two years).
+ Opthalmologic exam, looking for keratoconus and cataracts (every two years).
+ Mommography (40 years; follow up every other year until 50, then annual).
+ General physical/neurological exam. Routine adult care.
+ Low-calorie, high-fibre diet. Regular exercise. Monitor for obesity.
+ Clinical evaluation of functional abilities (consider accelerated ageing); monitor loss of independent living skills.
+ Neurological referral for early symptoms of dementia: decline in function, memory loss, ataxia, seizures and incontinence of urine and/or stool.
+ Monitor for behavioural/emotional/mental health.

Autism

Autism is one of the five pervasive developmental disorders (PDD) that are characterised by widespread abnormalities of social interactions and communication, severely restricted interests and highly repetitive behaviour (Volkmar et al 2005).

Characteristics of autism:

+ Inability to relate socially
+ Intense resistance to change
+ Fascination with objects

- Muteness or abnormalities of language
- Narrow interest
- Imposition of repetitive routine on self and others
- Good grammar and vocabulary, but inappropriate use of speech (Kanner 1943, cited in Dodd 2005).

Triad of impairments

Autism affects a person's ability in the three areas illustrated in Figure 3.12. These three areas are the core features of autism and are known as the triad of impairments.

Figure 3.12: Triad of autism impairments

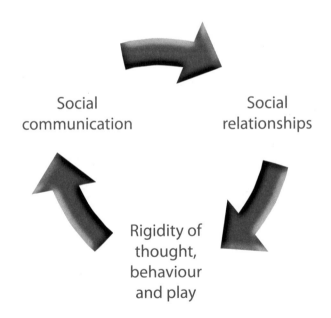

Source: Wing and Gould (1979), cited in Dodd (2005).

Pervasive developmental disorders (PDD)

This refers to a group of five disorders characterised by delays in the development of multiple basic functions, including socialisation and communication.

- Pervasive developmental disorder not otherwise specified (PDD-NOS)
- Autism
- Asperger's syndrome
- Rett syndrome
- Childhood disintegrative disorder (CDD)

Asperger's syndrome

Asperger's syndrome is characterised by milder symptoms that affect social interaction and behaviour. Language development is usually not affected. However, they often have problems in certain areas of language, such as understanding humour or figures of speech (for example, 'it's raining cats and dogs').

People with Asperger's syndrome have the intelligence to cope in society, but they often do not have the emotional resources to cope with the demands of everyday life (Dodd 2005). Some have particular skills in areas that require logic, memory and creativity, such as maths, computer science and music.

Pervasive developmental disorder – not otherwise specified (PDD-NOS)

Individuals with PDD-NOS have social deficits similar to autism and may have additional fundamental disturbances in communication, social behaviour, emotional regulation, cognition and interests. The symptoms arise during the first years of life, yet their severity or scope do not meet the more restrictive criteria for the PDDs (Volkmar et al 2005).

Most children with PDD-NOS have milder symptoms than children with an autistic disorder.

Basic principles of support and management of persons with autism

- Consistency
- Encourage participation
- Provide clear instruction
- Use visual aids
- Positive reinforcement
- Plan for success
- Prioritise (Dodd 2005)

The main goals when treating children with autism are to lessen associated deficits and family distress and to increase quality of life and functional independence. No single treatment is best and treatment is typically tailored to the child's needs (Volkmar et al 2005).

Some adults with autism spectrum disorder (ASD) may also have difficulty finding a job because of the social demands and changes in routine that working involves. However, they can get support to help them find a job that matches their abilities and skills.

Autism is often referred to as a hidden disability because people who are on the autistic spectrum show no significant physical differences to their peers. Rather, it is their behaviours that mark them out as different (Volkmar et al 2005).

Challenging behaviour

Challenging behaviour (CB) is behaviour of such intensity, frequency or duration that the physical safety of the person or others is placed in serious jeopardy or behaviour which is likely to seriously limit or deny access to the use of ordinary community facilities (Emerson 2001).

People with challenging behaviour are often seen as undesirable people to work with. Labels such as 'challenging', 'out of control' and 'violent' are often used to describe the individual. A person may display behaviours that challenge us, but the person should not be deemed or labelled challenging.

Unfortunately, these are the kinds of stereotypes that surround this group of people. Many people with challenging behaviours are misunderstood. When their behaviour is analysed and assessed, the trigger or function of the behaviour is established. One of the most common causes of CB is lack of effective communication.

Every person displaying such behaviours is different and the behaviours they display are not the only aspect of their personalities. It is imperative when working in this area that a positive mindset is maintained, as a pessimistic attitude can often be self-fulfilling.

Figure 3.13: Key causes/triggers of challenging behaviour

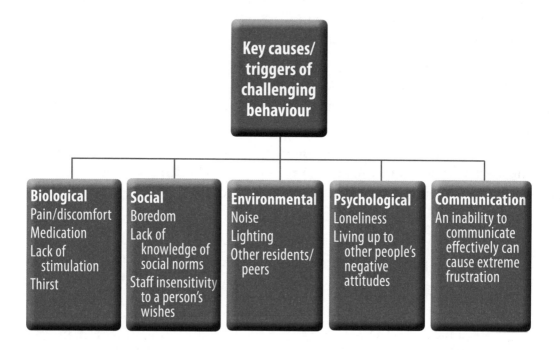

Assessment and functional analysis of behaviour are essential to determine the cause or trigger. It is essential to determine this first before attempting to modify a person's behaviour.

Types of challenging behaviour

+ **Self-injurious behaviour:** Hitting, head butting, biting.
+ **Aggressive behaviour:** Hitting others, spitting, kicking.
+ **Inappropriate sexualised behaviour:** Inappropriate touching.
+ **Destruction of property:** Throwing objects, turning over furniture.
+ **Other:** Faecal smearing.

Positive reinforcement

Positive reinforcement is a concept first described by psychologist B.F. Skinner in his theory of operant conditioning. Positive reinforcement is anything that follows a behaviour that makes it more likely that the behaviour will occur again in the future.

Reinforcement of challenging behaviour will contribute to the person's learning history by increasing the probability of such behaviour occurring in the future in response to similar motivational and environmental conditions (Emerson 2001).

The following scenario is adapted from Emerson (2001). It breaks down the above statement into a practical application.

A young man with a severe intellectual disability is feeling hungry. He is sitting in the living room of his community residence. (Environmental context) *He would like something to eat.* (Motivational state: food becomes established as positive reinforcer) *He does not have the ability or the opportunity to prepare his own food. A staff enters the room with tea and a biscuit for herself. As a result of previous learning* (learning history), *the man cries and bites his hand. The staff guesses that the man is communicating that he is hungry and brings him a biscuit* (positive reinforcement: delivery of food).

Inappropriate behaviours can be learned and can bring rewards. It is possible to teach people new behaviours to achieve the same aims.

Positive behaviour support

'Positive behaviour support (PBS)' is a general term that refers to the application of positive behavioural interventions and systems to achieve socially important behaviour change (Sugai et al 1999).

Positive behaviour support is a system to understand what maintains an individual's challenging behaviour. Behaviours that challenge are difficult to modify because they are functional. These behaviours are often supported by reinforcers within the environment. Caregivers in the person's environment have a tendency to reinforce his or her undesirable behaviours because the person will receive objects and/or attention because of his or her behaviour (Sugai et al 1999).

Functional behaviour assessment

- Describes a behaviour
- Identifies the contexts that predict when behaviour will occur
- Identifies consequences that maintain the behaviour.

Positive behaviour support processes involve goal identification, information gathering, hypothesis development, support plan design, implementation and monitoring (Tobin and Sugai 2005).

Importance of positive behaviour support

* Challenging behaviour can seriously affect a person's quality of life.
* It affects a person's ability to participate in community, which can lead to loneliness and low self-esteem.
* Accidental injury is a common medical issue in people who display aggressive behaviour.
* It can greatly limit a person's opportunities to integrate into society.

SUMMARY

This chapter examined the various aspects of disability and looked at the most common manifestations of each type of disability. People with disabilities are no different to anyone else in their desire to succeed and lead happy, fulfilled lives. To quote Joanne O'Riordan, 'I never look at myself as being different, I look at my life and say I'm unique' (www.journal.ie 2012). It is this uniqueness that should be celebrated and supported. It is only through this mindset and approach that disability service provision will change and evolve in the future.

REFERENCES

Appleton, R and. Marson, A. (2009) *Epilepsy*, 3rd edition, Oxford: Oxford University Press.

Bingham, E. (2011) 'Care of older people with epilepsy', *Nursing Older People*, 23(1).

Bjorklund, R. (2007) *Cerebral Palsy*, New York: Marshall Cavendish Corporation.

Boucher, J. (2009) *Autistic Spectrum: Characteristics, Causes, Practical Issues*, London: Sage Publishing.

Bull, M.J. (2011) 'Health supervision for children with Down syndrome', *Pediatrics*, 128(2), 1 August, pp. 393–406.

Carr, J. (1995) *Down's Syndrome Children Growing Up*, Cambridge: Cambridge University Press.

Corker, M. (1998) *Deaf and Disabled or Deafness Disabled: Towards a Human Rights Perspective*, Dublin: Open University Press.

CSO (2008) *National Disability Survey: First Results*, Dublin: Stationery Office.

Devinsky, O. (2007) *Epilepsy: Patient and Family Guide*, 3rd edition, New York: Demos Health.

Dodd, S. (2005) *Understanding Autism*, NSW: Elsevier.

Emerson, E. (2001) *Challenging Behaviour: Analysis and Intervention in People with Severe Intellectual Disabilities*, Cambridge: Cambridge University Press.

Fernyhough, C. (2005) 'What's on your mind?', *The Guardian*, 15 October, p. 22.

Gates, B. (2003) *Towards Inclusion*, 4th edition, London: Church Livingstone.

Gates, B. and Barr, O. (2009) *Oxford Handbook of Learning and Intellectual Disability Nursing*, Oxford: Oxford University Press.

Government of Ireland (2005) Disability Act, Dublin: Stationery Office.

Holt, R.I.G., Cockram, C. and Flyvbjerg, A. (2011) *Textbook of Diabetes*, Oxford: Wiley-Blackwell.

HSE (2011) *Time to Move on from Congregated Settings: A Strategy for Community Inclusion*, Report of the Working Group, Dublin: Stationery Office.

Hyde, A., Lohan, M. and McDonnell, O. (2004) *Sociology for Health Professionals in Ireland*, Dublin: Institute of Public Administration.

Jacobsen Bosch, J. (2003) 'Clinical practice: Health maintenance throughout the lifespan for individuals with Down syndrome', *Journal of the American Academy of Nurse Practitioners*, 15(1), pp. 5–17.

Krigger, K.W. (2006) 'Cerebral palsy: An overview', *American Family Physician*, 73(1).

Levitt, S. (2010) *Treatment of Cerebral Palsy and Motor Delay*, 5th edition, Oxford: Wiley-Blackwell.

Matthews, D., Beatty, S., Dyson, P., King, L., Meston, N., Pal, A. and Shaw, J. (2008) *Diabetes*, Oxford: Oxford University Press.

Sardegna, J. et al (2002) *The Encyclopaedia of Blindness and Vision Impairment*, 2nd edition, New York: Facts on File Inc.

Selikowitz, M. (2008) *Down Syndrome*, 3rd edition, Oxford: Oxford University Press.

Shorvon, S. (2009) *Epilepsy*, Oxford: Oxford University Press.

Shorvon, S. (2010) *Handbook of Epilepsy Treatment*, 3rd edition, Oxford: Wiley-Blackwell.

Silvers et al (1998) *Disability, Difference, Discrimination: Perspective on Justice in Bioethics and Policy*, Maryland: Rowman & Littlefield Publishers Inc.

Smith, D.S. (2001) 'Health management of adults with Down syndrome', *American Family Physician*, 64(6), pp. 1,031–8.

Sugai, G., Horner, R., Dunlap, G., Hieneman, M., Lewis, T., Nelson, C., Scott, T. and Liaupsin, C. (1999) *Applying Positive Behavioral Support and Functional Behavioral Assessment in Schools: Technical Assistance Guide*, U.S. Department of Education, Office of Special Education Programs, Centre on Positive Behavioral Interventions and Support.

Tobin, T.J. and Sugai, G. (2005) 'Preventing problem behaviors: Primary, secondary, and tertiary level prevention interventions for young children',*Journal of Early and Intensive Behavior Intervention*, 2(3), pp. 125–44.

Urbano, R.C. (2010), 'Health issues among persons with Down syndrome', *International Review of Research in Mental Retardation*, 39.

Van Dyke, D., McBrien, D., Siddiqi, S., Petersen, M. and Harper, D. (1997) 'Issues in health care for the adolescent and young adult with Down syndrome', International Research Conference on Down Syndrome, National Down Syndrome Society, Jacksonville.

Volkmar, F.R., Paul, R., Klin, A. and Cohen, D. (2005) *Handbook of Autism and Pervasive Developmental Disorders*, 3rd edition, New Jersey: John Wiley & Sons Inc.

Watson, D. and Nolan, B. (2011) *A Social Portrait of People with Disabilities in Ireland*, Dublin: Department of Social Protection.

WHO (2011) *World Report on Disability*, Malta: WHO.

WHO (2012) 'Deafness and hearing impairment', Fact sheet no. 300, World Health Organisation, available online at www.who.int.

Woodward, S. and Waterhouse, C. (2009) *Oxford Handbook of Neuroscience Nursing*, London: Oxford University Press.

Web sources:

- Brainwave – The Irish Epilepsy Association: www.epilepsy.ie
- Contact a Family: www.cafamily.org.uk
- DeafHear: www.deafhear.ie
- National Disability Authority: www.nda.ie
- National Down Syndrome Society: www.ndss.org
- National Health Service: www.nhs.uk
- World Health Organisation: www.who.int

4
Equality and Disability

INTRODUCTION

Many oppressed groups are stereotyped, which can be used as a mechanism to reinforce oppression. Stereotyping can also be described as labelling. Once a person or group is labelled, it can be difficult to change how they are perceived. This chapter will complement your understanding of disability awareness, introducing concepts of prejudice and labelling, conscious and unconscious discrimination, prejudiced language, legislation and anti-discriminatory practice.

KEY TERMS

- anti-discriminatory
- attitudes
- barrier
- disempowerment
- equality
- exclusion
- inclusion
- labelling
- marginalisation
- minority
- prejudice
- stereotyping

DISABILITY AND SOCIAL EXCLUSION

Disability and Social Inclusion in Ireland (Gannon and Nolan 2005) provides a valuable and necessary opportunity to explore the interface between poverty and inequality and the experiences of people with disabilities. This report confirms that extensive inequality exists in Ireland for those living with disabilities.

+ 38% of adults reporting a longstanding or chronic illness or a disability in 2001 were found to be at risk of poverty – more than twice the rate for other adults.

+ It also identified particular disadvantages for people with disabilities in relation to educational status, earnings and social participation.

+ 40% of those reporting a longstanding or chronic illness or a disability were in employment, compared with an employment rate of close to 70% for other adults of working age.

Disability can take many forms, e.g. restrictions in physical abilities, impaired vision or hearing, intellectual disability or mental health conditions. Under the Disability Act 2005, disability is defined as 'a substantial restriction in someone's capacity to work or take part in social or cultural activities due to a continuing physical, sensory, intellectual or mental health impairment'.

It is essential that all those who work with people who have disabilities consider their own personal values and prejudices. Unfortunately, we are not always aware of our prejudices, which may influence the way we view people and how we care for them.

Ireland is a member state of the United Nations, the European Union and the Council of Europe (including the Partial Agreement in the Social and Public Health Field). Irish legislation is therefore directly influenced by recommendations and legislation at an international level.

The National Disability Strategy (2004) includes a number of sectoral plans. This was considered to be a key measure taken by the government to ensure that people with disabilities can fully participate in Irish society. The outline of sectoral plans from the Department of the Environment, Heritage and Local Government highlights that within six months of the approval of the plan by the Oireachtas, each local authority will carry out an access audit of all public buildings, public parks, amenities and open spaces, roads and streets, pavements and pedestrian crossings, heritage sites, public libraries, polling stations and harbours within its control and identify what remedial action is necessary to make these buildings, etc. accessible for people with disabilities.

Furthermore, under the Programme for Prosperity and Fairness Agreement, the government made a commitment that all public services would be made more accessible. The Excellence through Accessibility Award is a joint initiative between the National Disability Authority and the Department of Justice, Equality and Law Reform.

The Disability Act 2005 is a positive action measure designed to advance and underpin the participation of people with disabilities in everyday life. It establishes a statutory basis for:

+ An independent assessment of individual health needs and educational services for persons with disabilities over age 18 years
+ Access to mainstream public services and actions to support access to public buildings, services and information.

Under part 3 of the Disability Act, public bodies, by law, must:

+ Ensure that people with disabilities can use their services easily and at the same location or access point as everyone else
+ Provide information in a way that suits the needs of people with disabilities – for example, by phone, by email, in plain English, large print or in Braille
+ Ensure that websites must meet specified accessibility standards
+ Ensure, where possible, that goods and services they buy or hire can be used by people with disabilities
+ Have accessible premises by 2015.

Despite this legislation, it seems that Ireland has quite a way to go towards ensuring equality for all. Inclusion Ireland, who are a voice for people with intellectual disabilities, reported in July 2012 that '153 young adults with an intellectual disability and/or autism leaving second level education will have no further education, training, or day service placement in September'. A statement in September 2012 by the same organisation highlighted the following:

The Programme for National Recovery early in 2011 undertook to ensure that 'the quality of life of people with disabilities is enhanced'. *Yet the budgetary measures implemented by Government to date have worsened their situation. Five successive years of cutbacks have undermined the independence of people with disabilities and diminished the supports they need to live ordinary lives, to enjoy individual autonomy and to participate in society as equals.*

ATTITUDES

One of the most important barriers to be aware of is attitude – both our own and those of others. Prejudiced attitudes can be obvious, hidden, secret or unconscious and can be hard to acknowledge. Prejudice is often applied by the more powerful over the less powerful through positions of authority.

A prejudiced attitude may be irrational, i.e. not based on reasonable, factual information. It is purely individual and often cannot be understood by another person. When working with people it is important to be aware of our own prejudices. This awareness can help minimise the risk of these prejudices leading to discrimination and potentially unfair treatment.

* Stereotyping can be a conscious or unconscious activity that is used to justify inequality and is an obstacle to the development of anti-discriminatory practice.
* Language can be used as a powerful tool to label people, thus perpetuating prejudice.
* Groups may be labelled as 'disabled', 'elderly', 'mentally ill', 'obese', etc.
* Individuals may be referred to through the condition they experience. For example, people with schizophrenia may be viewed as dangerous or people with autism as being challenging. A survey of attitudes to mental illness (HSE 2007) found that in relation to people who are perceived to be suffering from mental health difficulties but not stereotyped as dangerous, 10% of respondents thought there may be 'something to fear' from people with this disability coming into the community.

It is essential that we use the correct tone of voice within care practice and to ensure that we avoid patronising the person or disempowering them through our language.

Figure 4.1: Prejudiced language

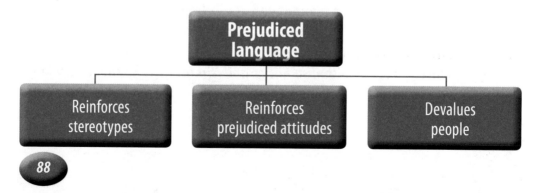

The effects of the denial of opportunities, disempowerment and stereotyping can all contribute towards creating marginalisation.

Figure 4.2: Discrimination

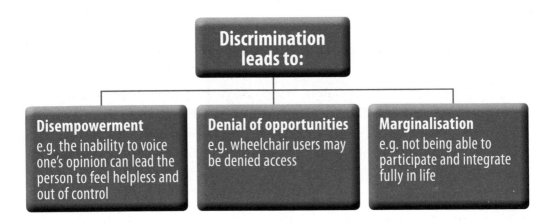

BARRIERS

Barriers may be **physical, legal, organisational** or **attitudinal**. Examples of barriers include the following.

- Steps are a physical barrier to wheelchair users.
- Legislation that sidesteps the real issues for people with disabilities.
- Lack of information about and the stigma surrounding mental illness create greater difficulties for those returning to work.
- Lack of accessible transport is a barrier to older adults and people who have a physical disability.
- Individual prejudices form a barrier for many individuals and groups, e.g. beliefs that people with disabilities create burdens that others have to bear.
- Institutional barriers occur when the very foundations of an organisation do not lend themselves to being inclusive, e.g. providing choices is too difficult because it is too expensive.

Task

1. Can you identify potential barriers a person with a disability may experience?

2. Can you suggest ways to remove the barriers experienced by people with disabilities?

The Employment Equality Acts 1998–2008 prohibit discrimination in recruitment, employment and training on nine grounds, including disability. Employers are legally obliged to provide employees with disabilities with reasonable accommodation to enable them to do their job, unless the cost would be disproportionate.

This Act provides for children with special education needs to attend a mainstream school with other students, unless this is not consistent with the best interest of the child or the effective provision of educational services for other children.

What is 'reasonable accommodation'?

Reasonable accommodation for customers with disabilities is described in the Equal Status Act 2000. It says that providers of goods and services must accommodate the needs of people with disabilities by:

making reasonable changes in what they do and how they do it where it would be very difficult or impossible for people with disabilities to obtain those goods or services without these changes unless those changes cost more than a nominal cost.

Under this legislation, public bodies must choose at least one member of staff as an Access Officer. The Access Officer helps or arranges help for people with disabilities to access public services. They might act as a point of contact for people with disabilities or they might set up systems to ensure that people with disabilities get the support they need.

PROMOTING EQUAL OPPORTUNITIES

Examples of initiatives that promote equal opportunities for people with disabilities include the following.

Work was undertaken by Cavan County Council and Kildare County Council with the support of the Equality Authority. A document, *Dara Has the Craic*, gives a timely and valuable account of initiatives taken at local authority level to embed a focus on accessibility for people with disabilities in planning, service design and service delivery. The emphasis was on 'how we do what we do' and how that could be adjusted to ensure equal access for people with all forms of impairment. In the words of one participant, seeing access for people with disabilities as 'an achievable, concrete, integral part of what we are doing anyway' eliminated the fear factor and neutralised any objections.

Another significant initiative was the creation of the Ability Awards through Kanchi (www.kanchi.org). This organisation was set up in 2000 by Caroline Casey. Kanchi promotes the value of people with disabilities in society and believes that the business community has the greatest capacity to lead the change.

Joanne O'Riordan, who is 16, was born with total amelia syndrome and has no limbs. Joanne advocates for people with disabilities to be treated like everyone else. Her engaging personality ensures that she is heard and over the last two years she has had a tremendous impact on our understanding of people with disabilities and what they 'can do' and how they can be helped to participate more in society. According to Joanne, as cited in the *Irish Times*:

> I want to live an independent life just like you. I don't want to live in the shadow of others because I want to make my own journey in life and I know if I'm given that chance I can and will succeed. I know that there must be someone out there in the world who can do something like this to make life much easier. It would not just help me, but indeed others who are in similar situations.

The Irish Paralympics team returned from the 2012 Paralympics Games in London with a total of 16 medals. This event has captured the imagination of the general public. It was a clear demonstration of the importance of inclusion and the contribution that individuals with disabilities can make to society.

Task

1. Make a list of inspirational people with disabilities and their contribution to society.

2. In April 2012, Joanne O'Riordan was invited to speak at the United Nations in New York at the International Telecommunication Union's conference, called 'Girls in Technology'. Read her speech at the end of this chapter.

PROMOTING EQUALITY IN CARE

HIQA states that their standards encapsulate a positive vision for the development of residential services to support people with disabilities in Ireland. They also state that this vision reflects the idea that 'what prevents people with disabilities from leading fulfilling lives is not lack of ability but other people's low expectations of them as embodied in some of the services provided for them'. With inspection of services for people with disabilities due to commence in 2013, it is essential that services promote equality within care settings.

- Strategies to promote equality should have objectives that are reviewed and evaluated and all objectives should have a timeframe.

- Every organisation should implement policies and procedures that can challenge negative behaviour, language and values constructively. These policies should be closely mapped to HIQA standards.

- Gestures towards inclusion, known as 'tokenism', should be avoided. Real commitment to promoting equality should be evident.

- Power relationships that may become established between the CCA and the person need to be recognised and monitored on an ongoing basis.

- Partnerships should be evident in every service.

- There should be a commitment to high standards of practice, sensitivity to language and promotion of positive images.

ANTI-DISCRIMINATORY PRACTICE

Anti-discriminatory practice can simply be deemed to be good practice. Anti-discriminatory practice is an approach that aims to reduce and ultimately eliminate the various forms of discrimination that may be encountered in care practice. It also involves challenging discrimination in others.

As with equal opportunities, there are many strands to anti-discriminatory practice. It involves the following elements.

+ Challenging discriminatory practice and discrimination within organisations.
+ Awareness of our personal prejudices and taking steps to overcome such prejudice.
+ Avoiding cultural stereotypes. It is important to gain an understanding of how individuals view their own religion and culture.
+ Helping people express a sense of pride in their identity.
+ Identifying the prejudices, stereotypes and assumptions that are used to devalue people and taking steps to counteract and eliminate such practice.

We can help to promote anti-discriminatory practice through the following.

Figure 4.3: Promoting anti-discriminatory practice

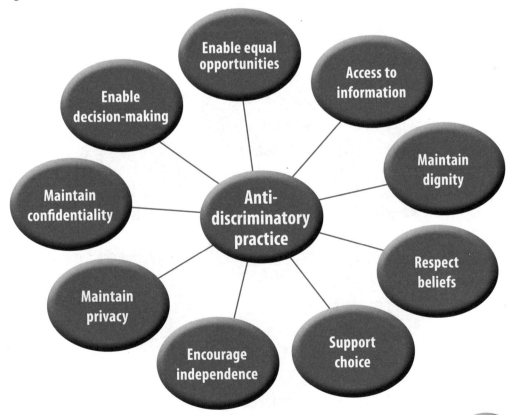

Specific strategies a care agency may use to promote anti-discriminatory practice within its own organisation might include:

* Ensuring everyone is involved in decision-making processes, e.g. advocacy groups, committees
* Ensuring food preferences, dietary requirements and hygiene requirements are chosen by the person using the service
* Allowing the person to choose which clothes they will wear
* Avoiding stereotypes
* Ongoing monitoring of equal opportunities policies
* Embedding issues related to equal opportunities into staff training
* Promoting care in a way that gives attention to a person's spiritual, social and cultural needs
* Having a policy to deal with discrimination.

Institutional discrimination can have a range of effects on an individual's personal identity and self-worth, including the following.

Figure 4.4: Effects of discrimination

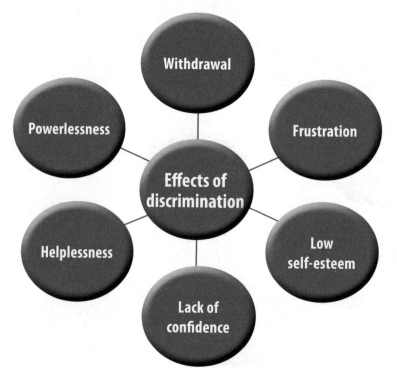

SUMMARY

In conclusion, disability must be understood in the context of society and how we as a society choose to include or exclude people with disabilities. It is essential that 'all means all'. We must work to ensure that people with disabilities can participate and enjoy life to the full.

Joanne O'Riordan is a 16-year-old teenager from Millstreet in Cork. She was born with a rare condition known as Total Amelia, meaning she has no limbs. Yesterday, she appeared before the International Telecommunication Union's conference 'Girls in Technology', receiving a standing ovation after delivering this keynote speech.

Good afternoon everyone! My name is Joanne O'Riordan and firstly I'd like to thank all of those at the United Nations and the people from the International Telecommunication Union for this amazing and unique opportunity to speak here in front of you today. Being invited to New York the week of my 16th birthday is simply unbelievable.

As you can see I was born without my limbs but my motto in life is, No Limbs No Limits. The disability I have is known as Total Amelia and it is one of the rarest conditions known to us. I believe there are only seven people in the world living with this physical form and furthermore there is no medical explanation as to why I was born this way.

However, my family and I have never allowed it to hold me back.

From an early age I have always relied on the use of technology to help advance my abilities. Be this in moving or communicating I developed an understanding of what I could achieve with technology from a young age.

I use technology in all aspects of my life, be it at home, in school or through the wider medium of interacting with others. My parents have told me that when I was one I first began to explore the use of technology with our old computer. I figured out how to use this software by simply moving my 'hand' and chin at a faster speed. Today I can type 36 words a minute and for someone with no limbs, I think that's an incredible achievement in itself.

The computer allowed me to play and follow certain games, which in turn helped me to learn my ABCs, maths and small words such as cat and dog. Needless to say, I'm a fiercely independent person but when I was born the technology that was there then was not as advanced as the technology we have now.

All my young life I've struggled and overcome barriers. I've surprised doctors, strangers, friends and even my own family by what I have achieved.

I must admit I'm always finding new ways or methods that would allow me to be the same as any other person. There is no such thing as 'normal' in my vocabulary. When I started school I, like all the other children, used my hand to write. I did this by putting my pen in between my shoulder and chin and as you can imagine this was an enormous challenge for me but I overcame the obstacle. I have always been breaking down barriers and overcoming obstacles. I do not look at the word Impossible and see it as Impossible. I look at that word and my life and say I'm Possible! Technology has made me even more determined to achieve a better standard and quality of life. I always think, if I can do this now, what would I achieve in the future?

Technology as we know is ever advancing and my question was soon answered when, at the age of seven, I started to develop a spinal condition known as scoliosis. This is a curvature of the spine. Unfortunately, this meant that I was not able to continue to write as I did and I had to find a new way of learning and developing my educational potential.

I'm very lucky that I have the support of my family, as they have never allowed anyone to hold me back. They have done everything in their power to ensure that I would not lose out on my education and technology was key in helping me.

A system was set up which allows my schoolbooks to be put on to CD. This in turn enables me to do all my work through a computer.

Nobody in Ireland has availed of this technology and I was extremely lucky to have a woman by the name of Christine O'Mahony helping me to make the process much easier. It took months to get the format right but when she did my life ultimately changed.

I now discovered that with one flick of my hand I was able to do all the things my other friends were doing with their fingers. I was able to be as good as them if not better. My quality of life has changed dramatically since I started using technology and only the other day I told my mother that technology is the limb I never had.

I can use my mobile phone, send texts, tweets, update my Facebook, play my PlayStation, Nintendo DS, iPad, iPod and laptop; without Microsoft, Adobe and Apple in my life I would not be doing and achieving my full potential. In fact I think my life would be quite different to what it is now. Believe it or not I simply use my upper and bottom lip, chin, nose and hand to work most if not all these systems.

Technology has opened up a world of possibilities, through which I have excelled in both my education and social environment around me. It is fair to say that I have been given the opportunities to grow, learn and adapt my lifestyle in a way that helps me, but I also know there are children and adults out there all over the world who do not have the same chances in life as I do.

I'm asking the Girls in Technology who are here today and who are the leading women within their field to start doing what I do, in my life: 'think outside the box'. Think of ways and means that you can make technology more accessible to those who really need it because let's face it, we all know women are better than men at most things so why not technology too?

It is my wish and it's my challenge to you and to others out there to build me a robot.

Yes, that's right, a robot! It sounds almost insane but as a child and even today I've always wanted and would love to have a robot. The main thing the robot would be doing is picking up the objects I drop, such as a pen, knife, fork or my phone.

This robot would become my hands and legs. So for example, if I was in the sitting room and I needed something from the kitchen, I would love for that robot to get me what I needed. I mean – to be fair – when you're lazy and sitting down most of you use a remote control because you're too lazy to get up and manually switch the TV over – and trust me that is lazy. So why can't I have a robot?

Call it crazy, call it insane, call it what you like – but the challenges I face every day get bigger and far greater to overcome. I know I can overcome these challenges but I need your help. I can't rely on my parents, my brothers, sister and others all my life. Can I? Certainly not and I don't want to!

I want to live an independent life just like you. I don't want to live in the shadow of others because I want to make my own journey in life and I know if I'm given that chance I can and will succeed. I know that there must be someone out there in the world who can do something like this to make life much easier. It would not just help me, but indeed others who are in similar situations. Life is about living and let's face it ladies, technology is not just a way of life, it's a way of living! And just because I have no limbs does not mean I will be limited. And neither should you!

Thank you!

Source: TheJournal.ie

REFERENCES

Equality Authority (2002a) *Disability Resource Pack: Positive Action for the Recruitment and Retention of People with Disabilities in the State Sector,* Dublin: Equality Authority.

Equality Authority (2002b) *Guidelines for Employment Equality Policies in Enterprises,* Dublin: Equality Authority.

Equality Authority (2002c) *Reasonable Accommodation of People with Disabilities in the Provision of Goods and Services,* Dublin: Equality Authority.

Equality Authority (2004a) *The Employment Equality Acts 1998 and 2004,* Dublin: Equality Authority.

Equality Authority (2004b) *The Equal Status Acts 2000 to 2004,* Dublin: Equality Authority.

Equality Authority (2005a) *Community Pharmacies Serving People with Disabilities,* Dublin: Equality Authority.

Equality Authority (2005b) *Guidelines for Equal Status Policies in Enterprises,* Dublin: Equality Authority.

Equality Authority (2007), *Dara Has the Craic,* Dublin: Equality Authority.

Equality Authority and the Library Council (2003) *Library Access,* Dublin: Equality Authority

Gannon, B. and Nolan, B. (2004) *Disability and Labour Market Participation,* Dublin: Equality Authority.

Gannon, B. and Nolan, B. (2005) *Disability and Social Inclusion in Ireland,* Dublin: Equality Authority.

Government of Ireland (2005) Disability Act 2005, Dublin: Stationery Office.

HSE (2007) *Mental Health in Ireland: Awareness and Attitudes,* Dublin: HSE.

National Disability Authority (2006) *Code of Practice on Accessibility of Public Services and Information Provided by Public Bodies,* Dublin: NDA.

Equality Organisations

* Accessibility.ie
* Equality Authority
* Inclusion Ireland
* Kanchi
* National Disability Authority

5
Understanding Mental Health

INTRODUCTION

This chapter will assist learners studying the Understanding Mental Health module. The chapter will consider current legislation and policy documents, the causes of mental illness, types of mental illness and treatments for mental illness. The chapter will also help learners develop a better understanding of the history of mental illness in Ireland. As is a common thread throughout this book, mental health will be considered across the six dimensions of health.

KEY TERMS

- asylums
- biological
- environmental
- existential
- functional psychosis
- humanism
- Mental Health Act
- neurosis
- organic psychosis
- psychological
- psychosomatic
- schizophrenia
- social approach
- statutory
- systematic approach
- voluntary

BACKGROUND

In the 1948 constitution of the World Health Organisation (WHO), health is defined as 'a state of complete physical, mental and social well-being, and not merely the absence of disease and infirmity'. This definition is useful insofar as it emphasises the fact that physical, social and mental factors are essential to health. However, the notion of always having complete physical, mental and social health is unrealistic and fails to recognise the importance of individual expectations and adaptability.

In 1984, WHO reviewed its definition of health and stated, 'Health is … seen as a resource for everyday life, not the objective of living; it is a positive concept emphasising social and personal resources, as well as physical capacities.' In 2007, WHO further defined mental health as 'a state of well-being in which every individual realises his or her own potential, can cope with the normal stresses of life, can work productively and fruitfully, and is able to make a contribution to her or his community'. Mental health, therefore, can be seen as a resource that allows us to function effectively in society, whereas mental ill-health is something that impedes normal human functioning.

Throughout history, mental illness and our understanding of it in society has changed. For over 100 years in Ireland, people who suffered from mental illness were locked away in asylums. However, records suggest that many people who were admitted to asylums had little reason to be there. People often ended up in asylums due to social inadequacy or because they were considered to be socially undesirable. These people were simply dumped by their communities into asylums to rid society of their presence. Criminals, epileptics and mentally ill people lived together in diabolical conditions. In the last decades of the asylums, psychiatrists tried to cure mental illness through the most barbaric methods. One of the most well-known institutions was the Monastery of St Mary of Bethlehem in London, which became known as 'The Bedlam'. People paid one penny to visit those incarcerated (who were held in chains and gags) in the asylum. The stigmatised view of the mentally ill stems from this time, and to this day, the word 'bedlam' means crazy and is used in everyday language throughout the UK.

The way in which people with mental health problems were treated in the past can affect our attitudes today. Mental illness still remains stigmatised and is viewed in society as a sign of weakness within the individual. If we think that someone is 'mad', then perhaps our response will still be that they should be locked up. People with mental health problems might not be 'locked up' today, but they can still be stigmatised and kept out of mainstream society.

According to Sheridan, as cited in Morrissey et al (2008), care for people with mental illness was influenced by the establishment of the Irish Free State, which rejected foreign practices and identified Ireland as distinctly Gaelic and Catholic. She argues that as a result, Ireland remained isolated from developments and changes in practices that were happening elsewhere in Europe.

By the 18th century, most asylums were in need of reform. Philippe Pinel is credited with pioneering reform in France. Pinel was put in charge of the Paris hospital system during the French Revolution. He removed the chains, created bright rooms and allowed the patients to exercise in the asylum grounds. The effect was instantaneous and order and peace began to prevail. During the 20th century there was an expansion in therapeutic methods of treatment, including the use of drugs. In the latter part of the 20th century, there was a movement towards care in the community and the dismantling of the large institutions.

Unfortunately, this early stigmatisation of mental illness has led to thought processes that may make younger generations reluctant to admit to feelings of anxiety and depression. Anxiety can begin in early childhood and develop across the lifespan. As people enter their teenage years, the challenges thrust upon them through physical development and additional environmental pressures, such as fitting into peer groups and establishing their own sense of identity, may lead to higher levels of anxiety that can eventually manifest as mental health difficulties.

Task

1. Consider a time in your own life when you felt stressed or unable to cope. Did you feel comfortable sharing these feeling with someone?
2. Look out for media articles about mental illness where stereotypes are perpetuated.

In 2007, the HSE National Office for Suicide Prevention (NOSP), in conjunction with voluntary and statutory sector partners, published research into mental health in Ireland in order to inform a national mental health awareness campaign (NOSP 2007). The report noted 11,000 episodes of deliberate self-harm presenting at hospital A&E departments each year (National Suicide Research Foundation) and up to 500 reported suicide deaths. The number of suicides rose to 527 in 2009, a 4% increase, and fell by 8% in 2010. On average, men are four times more likely than women to take their own life.

There were three key areas for action highlighted in the report: education around mental health and mental health problems; awareness and understanding of personal mental health; and recognising the importance of social and professional support. In recent years, we have seen the development of important policy documents on mental health – *Reach Out* (Health Service Executive et al 2005) and *A Vision for Change* (Government of Ireland 2006) – on suicide prevention. A fundamental principle underlying these policy documents is the development of whole-population approaches to mental health.

The Mental Health Act 2001 has been fully implemented since 1 November 2006. The Mental Health Commission and the Inspector of Mental Health Services have been in operation for a number of years. This Act provides for, among other things, rules about admission to psychiatric hospitals and rules about the rights of psychiatric patients.

If a person is involuntarily admitted to an approved psychiatric centre, they are entitled to:

- Have all decisions made in their best interests
- Be examined by a psychiatrist in the centre
- Be provided with certain information
- Have their retention reviewed by a tribunal
- Appeal to the courts in certain circumstances.

The Mental Health Commission has been in existence since 2002. Its main functions are to protect the interests of people who have been involuntarily admitted to an approved centre and to promote, encourage and foster the establishment and maintenance of high standards and good practices in the delivery of mental health services. The principal consideration, which applies when any decisions under the Mental Health Act 2001 are being made about the care and treatment of a person, is the person's best interests, with due regard being given to the interests of other people who may be at risk of serious harm if the decision is not made.

People who are being admitted or to whom treatment is being administered must be given an opportunity to express their views and have those views taken into account as far as is practicable. Programmes may be run by statutory, voluntary and independent or private organisations.

- **Statutory organisations** are funded through taxation, e.g. HSE services.
- **Voluntary organisations** rely on voluntary contributions from the general public for funds. They may receive grants from the government or from other agencies, e.g. the National Lottery Fund. Invariably these organisations are registered as charities. Examples in Ireland include Aware, Bodywhys, Console, Grow, Samaritans, Schizophrenia Ireland and Shine.
- **Private organisations** receive direct payment from the people who use the service. Examples include Highfield Private Hospital and St Patrick's Hospital in Dublin.

The above organisations may also combine efforts to provide a more comprehensive and effective programme for the service user or group.

Programmes may be located in hospitals, rehabilitation centres, community health centres, social work departments, schools and workplaces. Programmes may also be delivered directly to the person's home by a visiting professional or volunteer or through the Internet. Media campaigns, through organisations such as Aware, have played a pivotal role in bringing the issue of mental illness into the public domain and have helped to de-stigmatise illnesses such as depression. Those involved in the care of people with mental illness include general practitioners, psychiatrists, specialised nursing teams, community nurses, social workers, occupational therapists and carers.

Health promotion campaigns also play an important role in the prevention of mental health difficulties. Sport, music and social groups within the local community help to prevent isolation, which can have a detrimental impact on those suffering with mental illness. Walking groups and local support groups, such as those run by Aware and Shine, can have a tremendously positive impact on the person experiencing mental illness. Recovery programmes run by organisations such as Grow are vital in supporting people after hospitalisation.

There is a growing recognition that mental health promotion should not only be targeted at the individual, but should also take the individual's social and cultural context into account. Flexible rather than rigid working arrangements in schools, colleges and the workplace, for example, may reduce the incidence of stress. The promotion of mental health is not a simple issue, however, as the factors that cause mental illness are complex. Since many factors can interact to cause mental ill-health, all of these factors need to be addressed in the promotion of mental health. Social and cultural approaches to mental health in Ireland will have to consider, for example, the effects of the recession on people's mental health.

CAUSES OF MENTAL ILLNESS

It is considered that mental illness may be caused by predisposition, physiological and biochemical make-up or personality type. Predisposition refers to genetic or familial traits that may predispose a person towards a disease. These are known as **intrinsic factors**. **Extrinsic factors**, which are better understood as external factors, include stress, work, family problems, loss, bereavement, drugs, physical illness, childbirth and old age.

There is no evidence that there is any one specific cause of mental illness. The causes are complex and can involve many of the above factors. Evidence currently available suggests that certain disorders may be caused by environmental factors, while other disorders may be the consequence of hereditary/familial factors. There may often be an interplay of environmental and genetic factors that trigger the onset of mental illness.

The systematic approach (microscopic)

This approach sees illness as the product of circumstances in which the person lives (i.e. resulting from personal interactions in a particular context). The family is seen as an important microsystem that can cause behaviour symptomatic of mental illness. Laing and Esterson (1964) showed how individuals exhibited bizarre behaviour as a result of oppressive family relationships and were then labelled 'mad' by their family.

The social approach (macroscopic)

This approach stresses much broader social factors than the systematic approach. It looks at labelling and the medical process as well as focusing on the influence of the family. According to the social approach, we need to look further than these areas to find the cause of mental illness. The following factors may contribute:

- Poverty
- Social isolation
- Mundane, repetitive work
- Overcrowding
- Stressful life events
- Unemployment
- Relationships based on rigid hierarchies.

The social approach helps to explain the social class and gender inequalities in mental as well as physical health. This approach also views the community and wider society as the appropriate means of dealing with mental health and mental illness.

Behaviours that may occur as a result of mental illness include:

- Wandering
- Absconding
- Aggression
- Inappropriate behaviour.

FRAMEWORK FOR DIAGNOSIS

Models of diagnosis that include symptom and condition are based on the medical model of care. Classification of mental disorders is based on two classification systems: *The Diagnostic and Statistical Manual of Mental Disorders* (DSM IV-TR) and the International Classification of Mental and Behavioural Disorders (ICD 10). The DSM is currently in its fourth edition and is the system most widely used across Europe. The ICD is currently in its tenth edition. The purpose of these classification tools is to create guidelines to assist in diagnosis.

The difficulty with any diagnostic system is that it can limit our understanding to some extent. It is essential that mental illness is understood through the context of the individual experience of the person. Mental health and illness should be seen as a continuum along which each individual will travel. The direction of travel and the position of the individual on the continuum at any time will depend on social, biological, environmental and psychological factors.

Figure 5.1: Continuum of mental health

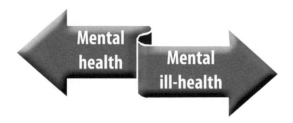

We should be aware that although medically and legally there is a need to classify certain disorders as 'mental illness', this can obscure the diversity of social, biological, environmental and psychological factors involved in a person becoming mentally ill.

It could be argued that labelling someone or a group of people as 'mentally ill' is unhelpful. The diagnosis of 'mentally ill' should not define the individual. Alzheimer's disease, anxiety, depression, post-traumatic stress syndrome, schizophrenia and stress are very different disorders.

Figure 5.2: Causal factors of mental illness

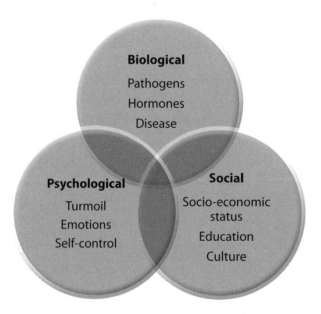

Three main models are used to help us understand mental health difficulties: biological, psychological and sociological. Together, they make up the biopsychosocial model.

The biopsychosocial model helps us understand the person through the interaction between the biological, psychological and sociological factors that cause illness. This model assumes that health and wellness may be caused by an interaction between these factors, i.e. the mind, body and environment interact to cause disease. Zubin and Spring (1977), as cited in Morrissey et al (2008), put forward the stress vulnerability model, which attempts to bring together all of the models when explaining the causes of schizophrenia. They suggest that each person has a degree of vulnerability, which may be determined by internal factors such as genetics, neuropsychological processes and factors such as traumas, disease and perinatal complications combined with life events and interaction with society.

We will consider the following three main categories of mental disorder: psychosis, personality disorders and neurosis (this is a general term for minor mental disorders, such as anxiety and depression).

Figure 5.3: The three main categories of mental disorders

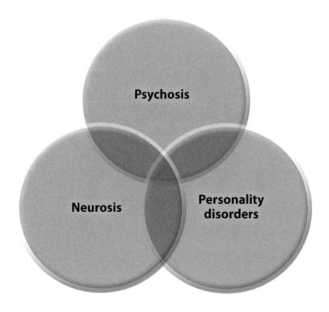

PSYCHOSIS

Figure 5.4: Organic and functional psychosis

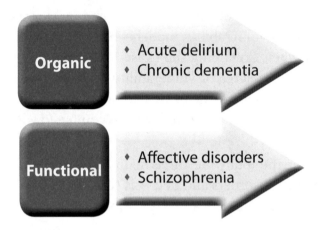

Organic psychoses

These are mental disorders that can be traced to an organic cause. They can be acute or chronic.

Acute conditions may be caused by brain tumours, infections, infectious diseases (usually temporary states of confusion), excessive drug, alcohol or substance abuse, food poisoning, hormonal disturbance, high temperatures, nutritional deficiencies or physical trauma. This temporary state is known as **delirium**.

Chronic psychoses are recognised as irreversible brain diseases causing memory and personality disorders, deterioration in self-care and hygiene, impaired cognitive ability and general disorientation.

Functional psychoses

This category includes schizophrenia and the affective disorders.

Schizophrenia

This is an umbrella term given to a group of psychotic disorders characterised by a distortion in rational thinking and behaviour. The signs and symptoms can include:

- Social withdrawal or withdrawal into a fantasy world
- Hearing voices (these are usually auditory hallucinations)
- The belief that thoughts are being controlled or heard by others (this is known as thought broadcasting)
- False beliefs about others or self (delusions)
- Inability to show emotions or inappropriate emotions
- Disordered speech with made-up words.

There are different kinds of schizophrenia, including acute, catatonic, childhood, disorganised and latent schizophrenia.

Affective disorders

These are characterised by extended and ongoing mood disturbances and distorted thoughts. The person may experience depression, mania and manic depression (otherwise known as bipolar disorder).

- **Mania** is described as a feeling of intense elation or euphoria. The person could appear intense and energetic but fails to achieve goals and lacks inhibitions (e.g. the person could go off on spending sprees).
- **Depression** is the reverse of mania. The person may present as sluggish, apathetic and with a total lack of motivation and may appear hopeless at times. The person may suffer from delusions or display agitation and negative feelings and become suicidal from time to time. Reactive depression is a response to an event that is prolonged and which may result in the person becoming mentally and physically exhausted.
- **Bipolar disorder or manic depression** is characterised by altering states of mania and depression, with the person swinging like a pendulum from one state to the other.
- **Anxiety:** The person can seem apprehensive due to feelings of fear of impending situations which may or may not be real. Symptoms include insomnia, irritability, lack of concentration, loss of appetite and nausea.
- **Phobias** are disproportionate fears that provoke a reaction that will seem irrational to others. The person may feel out of control and will do almost anything to avoid the fear.

PERSONALITY DISORDERS

Personality disorders are defined as persistent disorders of the mind that may cause the person to present with aggressive or irresponsible conduct. There are a range of different types of personality disorder, including psychopath and sociopath. Symptoms will include insensitivity to others, impulsive behaviour and a continual need for excitement. It is possible that the person will not express any guilt for their anti-social actions and their behaviour may not be changed by experience or punishment.

Invariably, they often cannot give or receive affection and find the demands of daily life difficult to cope with. A loss of touch with reality is often evident, leading the person into situations that place them at odds with society. Studies demonstrate that those with this diagnosis have experienced a difficult and tumultuous upbringing.

NEUROSIS

Depression

Depression may be described as 'feeling sad'. People who experience low mood from time to time do not experience clinical depression. However, a low mood is a snapshot of the experience of depression. People who are depressed see no end in sight. They may express feelings of hopelessness and low energy combined with low motivation to eat and socialise with other people. Sometimes this condition is prolonged and causes deep despair. It is essential for the person with depression to engage in treatment to aid recovery. There are different types of depression. These include reactive neurotic/exogenous, psychotic/endogenous and post-natal depression.

Depression in general can have the following effects.

Table 5.1: Effects of depression

Mental	Physiological	Social
Poor concentration	Tiredness	Avoidance of others
Impaired memory	Sleep disruption	Wanting to stay in bed
Slow and impoverished speech	Loss of appetite	Provide poor company so others avoid the
Sluggish thought processes	Weight loss	individual, which can
Depressed mood	Slowness of pace when walking	compound feelings of
Apathy	Stooped posture	worthlessness
Depersonalisation	Restlessness/tearfulness	
Suicidal ideas	Constipation	
Hopelessness		
Guilt		
Poor self-image		
Anxiety		

THE HUMANISTIC MODEL OF UNDERSTANDING MENTAL HEALTH AND ILLNESS

This approach to behaviour emerged in the 1950s, mainly through the work of Abraham Maslow and Carl Rogers. Humanistic theories share the following four characteristics.

- There is a **holistic** emphasis, i.e. the whole person is the focus of study. This is seen to be more important than the study of individual psychological processes.

- It is a **phenomenological** approach. This means that rather than analysing behaviour from the outside, behaviour is understood from the unique point of view of the person himself or herself. It is important to be aware of how the individual experiences their own world and also their self-awareness.

- Humanistic theory also has an **existential** perspective. Existence is not just about being alive. We must have a conscious awareness of what it means to exist – we are aware of the passage of time and that we are part of this process. We are aware of existing inside ourselves and of being separate from other people.

+ There is an emphasis on **personal agency**. People are seen to have free will and the capacity for change. It is important to understand that the person must play a role in their own recovery.

According to humanistic theories, we ourselves are largely responsible for what happens to us. As human beings, humanistic theory suggests that we are striving for growth, dignity and self-determination. Maslow suggested that people have a hierarchy of needs. Basic physical and safety needs have to be at least partially met to allow higher social and self-esteem needs to develop. The aim is to be the best we can be. This is what is known as **self-actualisation** (see Figure 1.2 on page 16).

The self-actualised person is sensitive to the needs and rights of others and strives to experience life to the full. They are not as concerned with social approval but have a clear sense of their own values and feelings. In short, they know and accept themselves and are in touch with their own personality.

Rogers (1961) suggested that an important influence in healthy personality development is **unconditional positive regard**. This can be thought of as a kind of acceptance from others. If parents and people who are important to us (significant others) communicate by words and actions that we are respected and loved regardless of what we say or do, then we have their unconditional positive regard. This allows us to develop high self-esteem and self-acceptance. If those around us only show us love and respect when we say and do what they want, then they are attaching **conditions of worth** to our relationship. Their acceptance is conditional on us getting into their scheme of things. This is known as **conditional love** and we feel that we must always struggle to be accepted.

Treatment approaches

Client-centred therapy (non-directive counselling) focuses on the wholeness of experience and emphasises a search for personal meaning. Behaviour and events are explored only from the point of view of the client. Rogers (1961) proposed three basic principles of the person-centred approach:

+ Genuineness (congruence)
+ Unconditional positive regard (warmth, acceptance, respect)
+ Empathy.

Task

Imagine you needed to talk to a care worker. What qualities would you like them to have? How would you like them to behave towards you?

This model emphasises the subjective experience of the individual; his/her personal views of the world and interpretation of events; and the individual's life in the here and now. Individuals are not victims of their desires or of their social circumstances. The individual can direct his/her own destiny and is responsible for the way in which life is lived.

Medical treatments (based on the medical model) include **anti-psychotic drugs** (also known as major tranquillisers or neuroleptics). They are used to relieve symptoms and help the individual to benefit from other forms of therapy, e.g. psychotherapy.

Anti-psychotic drugs can be used to control the more obvious symptoms of schizophrenia, including hallucinations and aggressive or agitated behaviour, by sedating the individual. The minimum necessary dosage to control symptoms is used because prolonged treatment with anti-psychotics can result in tardive diskinesia. This condition is characterised by involuntary muscular movements, spasms, twitches and tremor. Although there is a risk of this side effect, it is important to continue with treatment even when the symptoms of schizophrenia disappear because it is the treatment that is controlling the symptoms and relapse may occur if treatment is terminated.

According to Morrissey et al (2008), there is no evidence to suggest that psychosocial interventions alone are effective. However, psychosocial interventions work well alongside pharmacological interventions and a combination of all of these approaches is considered the most effective.

Table 5.2: Psychosocial interventions

Psychological	Social
Cognitive behaviour therapy Symptom reduction Stress reduction	Employment/education Social skills training Life skills training Social inclusion Functional improvement Well-being and quality of life
Family interventions	**Educative**
Psycho-education Communication training Problem solving	Relapse prevention Medication management/concordance Health promotion

Source: Morrisey et al (2008).

Task

1. Consider what it might be like to experience mental illness if you had (a) a sensory impairment or (b) a physical disability. What might impede your recovery?
2. How could you support a person with particular physical impairments/disabilities? You might want to consider your answer through the dimensions of health.

SUMMARY

This chapter has illustrated the history of mental illness in Ireland and demonstrated the continuum of mental health, identifying some common conditions and their signs and symptoms as well as identifying a range of treatments and strategies for meeting individuals' needs.

REFERENCES

Corry, M. and Tubridy, A. (2003) *Going Mad*, Dublin: New Leaf.

Department of Health and Children (2001) The Mental Health Act, Dublin: Stationery Office.

Government of Ireland (2006) *A Vision for Change: Report of the Expert Group on Mental Health Policy*, Dublin: Stationery Office.

Gross, R. (2005) *Psychology: The Science of Mind and Behaviour*, London: Hodder Arnold.

Health Service Executive (HSE), National Suicide Review Group and Department of Health and Children (2005) *Reach Out – National Strategy for Action on Suicide Prevention 2005–2014*, Dublin: HSE.

Health Service Executive (HSE) (2006) *National Office for Suicide Prevention Annual Report (2005)*, Dublin: HSE.

Laing, R.D. and Esterson, A. (1964) *Sanity, Madness and the Family*, London: Tavistock Publications.

Morrissey, J. et al (2008) *Psychiatric/Mental Health Nursing: An Irish Perspective*, Dublin: Gill & Macmillan.

NOSP (2007) *Reducing Suicide Requires a Concerted Collective Effort from All Groups in Society*, Dublin: National Office for Suicide Prevention.

Rogers, C. (1961) *On Becoming a Person*, London: Constable & Robinson.

World Health Organisation (WHO) (1992) *The ICD-10 Classification of Mental and Behavioural Disorders: Clinical Descriptions and Diagnostic Guidelines*, Geneva: WHO.

Websites

- Aware: www.aware.ie
- Bodywhys: www.bodywhys.ie
- Citizens Information: www.citizensinformation.ie
- Department of Health: www.dohc.ie
- Grow: www.grow.ie
- Health Service Executive: www.hse.ie
- Shine: www.shineonline.ie

6
Therapeutic Communications: Knowledge for CCAs

INTRODUCTION

This chapter will enhance your understanding of the importance of communication when working with individuals in receipt of care services. It is essential that community care assistants (CCAs) not only understand the importance of their own interactions in care work, but also the importance of written and documented communication within the care setting.

KEY TERMS

- accountability
- advocacy
- assessment
- attributes
- care plan
- confidentiality
- core values
- documenting
- empathy
- empowerment
- reflect

PROFESSIONAL CARING RELATIONSHIPS

'Across time and settings, people everywhere have subscribed to the view that close, meaningful ties with others is an essential feature of what it means to be fully human' (Ruff and Singer 2000: 31, as cited in Hargie and Dickson 2004).

The professional caring and helping relationship is different from the personal relationships we have in our lives. The quality of a professional caring relationship can have a profound effect on individuals and on the individual's perceptions and experience of receiving care services. It is imperative, therefore, that all professional caring relationships are underpinned by the core values and principles that are essential to successful care work. Professional CCAs need to develop their interpersonal skills and knowledge in order to be effective helpers. They also need to develop self-awareness through reflective practice and should be supported and supervised to carry out their professional role. A positive professional caring relationship, although sometimes temporary, can significantly improve the quality of life for the individual and bring enormous satisfaction for the CCA.

Task

How is a working relationship with a vulnerable individual different from an everyday personal relationship?

Sometimes it is mistakenly assumed that because we live in a social world where people interact with others all the time, work with people can be done by anybody. The key ingredients to being a good CCA are a positive outlook, a cheerful disposition and the capacity to convey warmth.

THE DIFFERENCES BETWEEN PROFESSIONAL AND PERSONAL CARING RELATIONSHIPS

Some of the ways professional caring relationships differ from personal caring relationships are shown in Figure 6.1.

Figure 6.1: The differences between professional and personal caring relationships

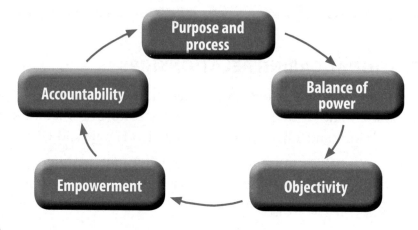

Purpose and process

Working with people requires carefully structured and decisive processes that are considered, purposeful, planned and systematically reviewed. It is expected that the CCA will relax, laugh and joke with colleagues and individuals in receipt of their care, but this will be in the context of work rather than in the context of personal relationships. It must be considered how this relationship is defined and what underpins the relationship.

Balance of power and objectivity

People who work together often do not choose each other. In a care setting, the workers and individuals relate to each other across a range of different situations and roles. If you found yourself in receipt of care, you would be aware that it is essential within this relationship that the person with whom you interact strikes a balance between being approachable and creating distance where necessary.

Empowering rather than helping

The task will be to enable or empower the individual. We aim to induce independence and ultimately be enabling towards the person we care for.

Accountability

We are accountable to our employer and our client. We must never forget that sometimes there is an imbalance of power between the CCA and the individual, which may lead to abuse. Occasionally, extreme examples of this abuse of power by CCAs are the focus of media attention. However, subtle and passive forms of the unconscious abuse of power can result in discriminatory, oppressive or abusive practice.

PROFESSIONAL CCAs

CCAs interact with a range of individuals, such as older adults, children and families, young people, people with a range of health problems, people with learning difficulties, people with physical disabilities, people with sensory disabilities, people with drug and alcohol problems and homeless people. CCAs also work in a range of health care and social care contexts, including residential, day care and home care settings.

ATTRIBUTES OF EFFECTIVE HELPERS

In order to be effective helpers, CCAs must possess a number of essential personal qualities and attributes (see Figure 6.2).

Figure 6.2: Attributes of effective helpers

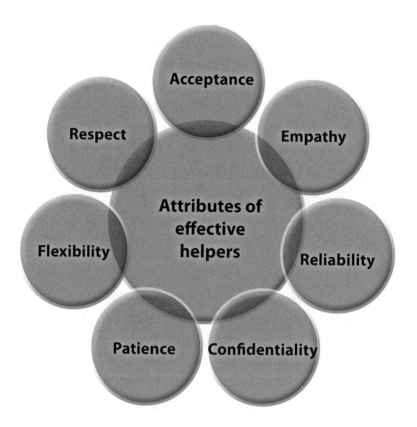

- **Acceptance:** As CCAs, we must recognise that all human beings are unique people worthy of respect. It is essential that we look beyond any outward behaviour or disability and accept the person as an individual, irrespective of their appearance or beliefs.
- **Empathy:** It is essential that we can enter the person's world and appreciate and understand how they are feeling.

- **Reliability:** CCAs need to be dependable and trustworthy.
- **Confidentiality:** CCAs must ensure that information about individuals is not passed on to other people outside the care setting without first consulting the individuals themselves. We should not discuss individuals with others and should only pass on private information on a need-to-know basis. (This issue will be considered further below.)
- **Patience:** We must be able to move at the individual's own pace.
- **Flexibility:** It is important to be able to adapt to different situations and to different people, including their different ways of working.
- **Respect for others:** We must be aware that all people have personal rights and the need for dignity and privacy. These rights and needs should be respected at all times.

EMPATHY

Empathy is understanding and experiencing how another person is feeling. It involves making a conscious effort to understand a person holistically and requires being able to convey this understanding to that person. In caring relationships, it is very useful to develop the skills of listening and responding empathically.

CCAs can develop empathy in their relationships with individuals. This will involve actively listening in order to understand what the individual is communicating and then clearly communicating back this understanding.

CONFIDENTIALITY

The right to confidentiality

Everyone has the right to confidentiality. As a CCA, you may experience more disclosure than anyone else. Frequently, confidential information is shared and you may have access to medical or social care records that often contain lifelong histories. In order to sustain a helping relationship, it is vital that individuals can trust their CCAs to maintain this confidentiality. Individuals must be able to talk freely and honestly. This is core to safeguarding the individual and to preventing abuse. CCAs should not discuss individuals they care for in public. If confidences are broken, the helping relationship and the trust that have been built up can break down, leading to significant difficulties for the individuals concerned, for employees and for service providers.

Handling confidential information

CCAs

It cannot be absolutely guaranteed that all information shared will be kept confidential. CCAs, therefore, may face some difficult situations regarding disclosure. There may be situations, for example, when it is necessary to share information with colleagues in order to be able to work effectively. There may even be situations where it is essential to share confidences, such as when vulnerable groups (for example, children or older people) need to be protected. All employers and organisations are required to have relevant policies and guidelines on confidentiality in place.

Students

When handling confidential information, students who have work placements in care settings need to adhere to the same general principles as professional CCAs. If students are writing case studies or other reports on individuals as part of their course, they need to ensure that all names and details are changed in order to protect identities. In classroom group discussions, individuals should be referred to indirectly and never by name. It is acceptable and essential that students share real-life situations throughout their training, as such sharing of information can enhance learning. However, it could occur in a learning situation that another student identifies a client if both students are working in the same service. If this situation arises, it is imperative not to make reference to this outside of the learning environment – what's said in the room stays in the room.

Another important point to note as a student and/or as an employee is to never discuss a client with colleagues, either in the workplace or outside of work. This is a clear breach of confidentiality and can lead to dismissal from employment.

Access to files

People have the right to know what has been recorded about them. Most information that is held in files may be accessed by the individual concerned.

Sharing information with other professionals

Sometimes it is necessary for an individual's well-being to share information with other professionals. These could be professionals within the same setting or professionals from a different setting. It will be necessary to pass on information during handover to ensure continuity of care. It may also be necessary to pass on information to the individual's GP if the need arises.

Safety of individuals

There are situations where confidential information about an individual needs to be passed on to other people in order to protect the safety of that individual. An example of this would be a young adult with mental health difficulties who lives in supported accommodation and who is threatening to commit suicide.

Safety of other people

Occasionally an individual may threaten to harm other people and action has to be taken to ensure that the other people are protected, e.g. a person might confide that they want to harm someone or a group of people.

Legal requirements

The Data Protection Amendment Act 2003 updated the 1988 Data Protection Act. This legislation implements provisions of EU Directive 95/46. The Acts set out the general principle that individuals should be in a position to control how data relating to them is used.

The Data Protection Commissioner is responsible for upholding the rights of individuals as set out in the Acts and for enforcing the obligations upon data controllers. The commissioner is appointed by the government and is independent in the exercise of his or her functions. Individuals who feel their rights are being infringed can complain to the commissioner, who will investigate the matter and take whatever steps may be necessary to resolve it. There are certain situations where there is a legal requirement to disclose information. For example, information regarding infectious diseases must be passed on to a public health doctor. If a person contracts Legionnaires' disease, it will be essential for this information to reach the relevant person in order to protect public health.

You must:

+ Obtain and process the information fairly
+ Keep it only for one or more specified and lawful purposes
+ Process it only in ways compatible with the purposes for which it was given to you initially
+ Keep it safe and secure
+ Keep it accurate and up to date
+ Ensure that it is adequate, relevant and not excessive
+ Retain it no longer than is necessary for the specified purpose or purposes
+ Give a copy of the individual's personal data to them upon request.

ATTITUDES AND ATTRIBUTIONS

All helping relationships in a care context are underpinned by our attributions. What we attribute to a situation will depend on our values and will incorporate how we:

+ Treat people
+ Maintain confidentiality
+ Are able to respect rights and choices
+ Adhere to anti-discriminatory practice.

Attributes of effective helpers are closely linked to interpersonal skills. Values in care work include preserving dignity, respecting people, encouraging independence, building self-esteem, empowering people, allowing self-determination and supporting acceptable risk-taking.

Where values are put into practice, they result in principles. Care work is informed by the principles of good practice. These are led by our own principles and values, which inform and lead to the development of policies, such as those that care providers have on the issues of confidentiality and equal opportunities. HIQA standards are informed by principles that lead to the development of local policy, thus creating good practice in a care setting.

A CCA's attitude and values can be observed by many aspects of his/her behaviour. It can be difficult to change attitudes and values, but in care work it is necessary to always try to apply the principles of good practice. Thus, it is essential that CCAs strive to:

* Be self-aware, i.e. identify their own prejudices and stereotypes of certain groups
* Respect and value individuality in people
* Promote each individual's rights, e.g. the right to choice, privacy, dignity, independence, confidentiality and protection.

Attitude will have a significant impact on our interactions. Katz and Stotland (1959), as cited in Hargie and Dickson (2004), consider attitude in terms of three constituent elements:

Cognitive – *contributing knowledge or beliefs about the target in question, which may be a person, object, event or any attribute of these;*

Affective – *reflecting how one feels about the target, either positive or negative in liking or disliking. For some, this is the most important attribute; and*

Behavioural – *having to do with one's predisposition to behave in a certain way towards the target.*

According to Hargie and Dickson (2004), the elderly are frequently subjected to simplified forms of speech that can seem patronising. In addition, negative stereotypes of older people appear to be at the bottom of this way of relating. Activating a stereotype may suggest incompetence, decline or senility and younger speakers may tailor what they are saying to these beliefs. Grainger (1995), as cited in Hargie and Dickson (2004), found that baby talk (BT) is a feature of CCAs' communication, often regardless of the level of competence of the receiver.

Gudykunst and Ting-Toomey (1996), as cited by Hargie and Dickson (2004), state that communication shapes culture. It is essential when communicating in a care setting that shared meanings are given careful consideration. In Ireland, increasing diversity in the CCA population over the past 15 years means greater attention must be given to this issue. While older populations remain largely a homogenous group within disability and mental health settings, we increasingly see more diverse populations emerging. It is imperative that we place some emphasis on the colloquialisms that emerge in settings and the differences in shared meanings.

Task

Consider colloquialisms/differences in communication and shared meaning that might emerge in any group setting in Ireland.

MOTIVATING SKILLS IN CARE WORK

An important interpersonal skill in care work is the ability to help motivate individuals. Many individuals are well motivated themselves, but others may require motivational skills from CCAs to help them develop the desire to act and behave in particular ways.

Motivation is about desire, interest and the drive to do or change something. In order to do anything, we must be motivated. Motivation provides the drive for human beings to achieve and regulate their behaviour. People are usually motivated through rewards and these are generally concrete and tangible, e.g. a CCA may be motivated to work competently and regularly in order to receive a wage (financial reward). Rewards that motivate actions and learning are often less tangible and may relate to areas such as self-esteem, status, happiness and achievement. For example, a person may be motivated to work in order to achieve social contact in addition to a monetary reward.

The energy, enthusiasm and commitment that CCAs bring to their care setting are crucial factors in helping individuals develop motivation. One of the consequences of being in residential care is that certain individuals may develop 'learned helplessness'. CCAs must work with each individual to try to find the rewards that will motivate behaviour and activity.

A study was carried out by Langer and Rodin (1976) on the effects of allowing personal decision-making amongst nursing home residents (in the care of a plant). 'The ability to sustain a sense of personal control in old age may be greatly influenced by societal factors, and this in turn may affect one's physical well being … more successful aging occurs when an individual feels a sense of usefulness and purpose' (Langer and Rodin 1976).

For this study, two floors of a nursing home were selected. On one floor, a group of residents was told that the staff would be there to help them at all times. Over a period of three weeks, 71% of this group showed signs of deterioration. On the other floor, where the group was encouraged to make decisions for themselves, the residents actually improved. These residents were more engaged in activities, more mentally alert and happier. The study concluded that 'a feeling of helplessness may contribute to psychological withdrawal, disease and death'.

EMPOWERMENT

Empowerment is all about giving people power so that they can make their own decisions about their own lives. In care work, individuals should be empowered to make their own choices and decisions. This is a shift away from how care work has been carried out previously. In the past, professionals were seen as the experts with all the power to make decisions about the kind of care service individuals would receive and the individual was nothing more than a passive recipient in the care process.

CCAs and organisations that work with the vulnerable have considerable power compared to the individuals who receive the care. Therefore, it is essential to make conscious and ongoing efforts to share power with individuals. At times this can prove very difficult, particularly with service users who are either unwilling or unable to make decisions and choices for themselves.

> *Any situation in which some men prevent others from engaging in the process of inquiry is one of violence … to alienate humans from their own decision making is to change them into objects. – Paulo Freire*

There are different models and approaches to empowerment, including:
- Giving or sharing power with the individuals
- Enabling the individuals to develop power
- Equal power between the individuals and worker.

Once there is equal power between a worker and an individual, the worker can take a step backwards, as the individual is then fully empowered. It is essential that we work with people through principles of empowerment. The HIQA Standards for Older People in Residential Settings and the draft standards for residential services for people with disabilities place an emphasis on autonomy, informed decision-making and consent.

The empowered CCA

CCAs must be empowered to make decisions, access resources and be aware of their own strengths and weaknesses. However, CCAs as a professional group remain undervalued, underpaid and undertrained. As a consequence, a proportion of CCAs are themselves disempowered and find it very difficult to empower others.

CCAs must be trained to the highest possible standards. This training should be both engaging and rewarding for the CCAs and not simply a compliance 'tick box' exercise. Employers should recognise the importance of training in care work and promote CCAs' efforts to educate themselves and update their skills, as a trained and competent care force will ultimately enhance the experience of the people who utilise their services. Training will become more and more essential if those in receipt of care services gain a role in choosing their services. Employers' initiatives to promote training and education amongst employees should be commended and recognised by those who fund services in order to continue to enhance the provision of care for all.

ADVOCACY

An advocate is someone who speaks up for people's rights, standing alongside an individual who is disadvantaged and speaking out on their behalf. According to HIQA Standard 17 Autonomy and Independence, it is essential that each resident can exercise choice and control over his/her life and is encouraged and enabled to maximise independence in accordance with his/her wishes.

Aims of advocacy

- Increase client control
- Overcome barriers that restrict opportunities
- Ensure appropriate service
- Protect human rights
- Ensure a better quality of life
- Respond to individual needs
- Orientate towards client outcomes

ESTABLISHING RELATIONSHIPS

The initial relationship between the CCA and individual may be a collaborative relationship when, broadly speaking, the individual welcomes the support of the CCA. Whatever type of relationship it is, the three core conditions first identified by Carl Rogers (1961) for creating a safe atmosphere that value the client are relevant.

Although Rogers proposed these conditions as a basis for counselling relationships, they have been found to be equally applicable in establishing all kinds of helping relationships. If CCAs demonstrate and apply these conditions in establishing relationships with individuals, then a positive working relationship is likely to be formed:

+ Unconditional positive regard (sometimes called warm acceptance)
+ Empathy (sometimes called understanding)
+ Congruence or genuineness (sometimes called sincerity).

ACTIVE LISTENING

Body language is vitally important when communicating with other people, so it is imperative that we adopt a body posture that will encourage interaction with the individuals we are helping. Egan (1990) proposed certain essential skills for showing that levels of attention are present during an interaction. He used the acronym SOLER to summarise these skills:

S Sit or stand so you are facing the person **SQUARELY**

O Maintain an **OPEN** or interested posture

L **LEAN** towards the person when they are speaking

E Maintain **EYE CONTACT** without staring

R Remain **RELAXED** during the conversation

In order to promote an effective interaction, you should:

+ Develop a good rapport
+ Foster a feeling of trust
+ Ensure you are in a comfortable environment

+ Ensure privacy
+ Remain focused on the person
+ Pace the conversation.

ESTABLISHING CONTRACTS

Positive working relationships can be more effective if some kind of contract between the CCA and the individual is agreed. This is an implicit and informal contract in which the CCA and individual identify what is expected of each of them in terms of behaviour and actions. In an equal and fully empowered relationship, this is established equally between the CCA and the individual. In some care settings and situations that are more formal, explicit written contracts are appropriate.

Sometimes contracts are essential for people who are living in a residential setting where the behaviour of an individual resident may be affecting all the other residents, making it essential to set boundaries. Contracts are always useful to clarify points and expectations about the helping process. Contracts reduce confusion, and as a result, misunderstandings are less likely to arise. The establishment of a contract ensures that everyone knows what is expected of them.

MAKING AN ASSESSMENT

Assessment is a key area of communication in care work. It is important when performing an assessment that we communicate and find out about the person at an in-depth level. It is essential that all assessment is 'needs led'. Whatever level of assessment is required, the most fundamental principle of needs-led assessment is to work *with* the individuals and their significant others. Some people will have informal carers who are crucial to their health and well-being. These carers are often family members but may also be friends and neighbours.

Figure 6.3: The assessment process

Clarify expectations to ensure the person understands the purpose, mechanism, timescale, possible outcomes and their rights and entitlements in the assessment process.

Assess needs by using appropriate methods, consulting with all relevant people and working towards as much consensus as possible. When the person is capable of expressing their opinions, these views must carry a lot of weight. It is then essential for the assessor and person to agree on the priority that each identified need should be given.

Assessment process

Promote participation to actively involve the person and their carers in the process. Some people will have a clear understanding of their needs, whereas others may be confused or unable to articulate their opinions or needs. It is important that assessors work to identify positives and strengths as well as difficulties and needs in a particular situation.

Record needs. All relevant parties, such as the individuals, carers, representatives of the person and other agencies involved in the assessment, should receive a copy of the assessment form. The assessment record will then inform and lead to the development of a care plan.

Whatever the level and scope of the assessment, it is always a two-way process between the person and the assessor. Sometimes other people, such as care professionals and agencies, will need to be involved. At the start of the assessment, it is helpful if the assessor uses good interpersonal skills to establish a relationship of trust. Then, all records should be:

* Confidential
* Structured
* Accurate
* Up to date
* Easy to read and understand.

THE CARE PLAN

A care plan is a plan that identifies the most appropriate ways to meet the needs of the individuals, as agreed in the assessment process. Resources have to be available to meet the needs and priorities have to be set with timescales and action points. Many individuals who have a care plan will have a range of different types of need. For many individuals, the care plan will comprise a combination of support, care, enabling, treatment and forms of intervention. For other individuals, the care plan will be much simpler and identified needs may be met by the provision of a single service.

CCAs must understand the importance of completing a care plan appropriately. Documentation refers to the action of writing or documenting your work. It may provide an account of your interactions with or observations of the person. It will enable other CCAs to respond to the needs of the person without having to repeat information on an ongoing basis. It may be utilised in legal proceedings and it has the capacity to become a legal document in the event of an action being taken in relation to a case. It will also:

- Identify needs and goals
- Keep a permanent record of events
- Inform others
- Enable accountability for all involved.

It is important to document the information obtained from the person or their family for effective communication. Always identify the ways in which the person's basic needs can be easily met and document how to calm the person down in the event of frustration due to unmet needs. Always make sure to maintain eye contact, use gestures when communicating, reduce distractions that may impede your ability to communicate, listen to the person and clarify understanding.

Figure 6.4: Barriers to communication

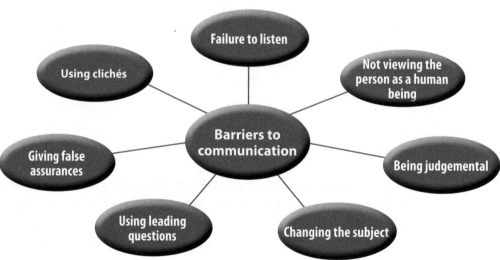

Source: Taylor, Lillis and Lemone (1997).

Obvious barriers to communication in a care setting include sensory loss and/ or other losses of function that may lead to difficulties. It is important that efforts are made to understand colloquialisms. In Ireland there are a range of dialects, particularly in rural areas, that require local knowledge. We must take time to develop an understanding of colloquialisms and ensure that we always have shared meaning when we are talking to people.

According to Zaretsky et al (2005), as cited in Hargie and Dickson (2004), impaired communication is the decreased, delayed or absent ability to receive, process, transmit and use a system of symbols. Impaired communication may be caused by expressive aphasia (the loss of ability to verbally express oneself) or receptive aphasia (the loss of ability to understand language).

Sensory loss can be a visual or a hearing impairment.

+ **Visual impairment** is a change in the amount or patterning of incoming stimuli, accompanied by a diminished, exaggerated, distorted or impaired response to such stimuli.

+ **Hearing impairment** is a change in the amount or patterning of incoming stimuli, accompanied by a diminished, exaggerated, distorted or impaired response to such stimuli. (See Chapter 3 for further information on this disability.)

Practical ways to assist will include asking the person about their hearing function. Be alert to how you communicate with the person in order for them to understand. You may notice that you have to speak louder, more slowly and distinctly. You may have to use gestures or bring the person to a quieter environment. While interacting with the person, observe and listen to his/ her attempts to communicate. If the person uses communication devices, encourage their use. Observe for the presence of non-verbal expressions, which may include blinking, hand squeezing or gesturing. For further information on ways to assist, refer back to Chapter 3.

SUMMARY

This chapter has focused on a range of important issues that arise when communicating and interacting in a care environment. This essential chapter, if followed, will lead to improved social interactions and shared understanding within the care environment.

REFERENCES

Egan, G. (1990) *The Skilled Helper: A Problem Management and Opportunity Approach to Helping*, 7th edition, California: Brooks/Cole Publishing.

Hargie, O. and Dickson, D. (2004) *Interpersonal Theory and Practice: Research Theory and Practice*, 4th edition, Sussex: Routledge.

HIQA (2009) *National Quality Standards for Residential Care Settings for Older People in Ireland*, HIQA.

Langer, E.J. and Rodin, J. (1976) 'The effects of choice and enhanced personal responsibility for the aged: A field experiment in an institutional setting', *Journal of Personality and Social Psychology*, 134, pp. 191–8.

Rogers, C. (1961) *A Therapist's View of Psychotherapy: On Becoming a Person*, London: Constable.

Taylor, C., Lillis, C. and Lemone, P. (1997) *Fundamentals of Nursing: The Art and Science of Nursing Care*, Sydney: JP Lippincott Company.

Websites

- Data Protection Commissioner: www.dataprotection.ie
- HIQA: www.HIQA.ie
- Pedagogy of the Oppressed: www.pedagogyoftheoppressed.com

7
Work Experience

INTRODUCTION

A work placement is integral to a number of vocational educational and training programmes, including the Community and Health Services Award. They are an excellent way of gaining experience of working within different sectors of health care, giving the community care assistant (CCA) an opportunity to explore the reality of working within different organisations with people with a variety of needs while integrating new learning in practice. Placements also enable a student to establish where their career preferences lie – there is nothing wrong with acknowledging and accepting that you have a preference for one type of work over another.

Experiential learning is important for CCAs, as experience will enhance and illuminate care practice. This chapter explores the role of a CCA as well as a wide range of skills and qualities that are necessary for working in health care. It encourages you to consider these aspects with a focus on your professional and personal development.

KEY TERMS

- advocacy
- community care assistants (CCAs)
- experiential learning
- formal and informal carers
- mentoring
- reflective practice

THE ROLE OF THE HEALTH CARE WORKER

Following on from the question of who needs care is the question 'who cares?' Not everyone can care on a formal basis, and not all CCAs can care for people with different needs. For example, while some CCAs enjoy working with older people, others prefer to work with children and vice versa; some people can work with people with mental health difficulties, whereas others prefer to work with people with learning disabilities. For a person in need of care, there can be little worse than being cared for by someone who either does not care or actually resents caring or resents caring for people within that specific sector. This is why it is so important for CCAs to carefully consider the role that they undertake and understand where they want to work.

WHO ARE INFORMAL CARERS?

At this point, it is necessary to include statistics about informal carers because an important part of the work of a care team is to provide support for informal carers.

The term 'informal carer' is given to someone who cares for a relative, friend or neighbour on a regular and frequent basis, usually in the person's own home. Informal carers and formal carers often carry out similar tasks, but carers are in paid employment, whereas informal carers are not paid. According to the 2006 census, there were 161,000 informal carers in Ireland and 65.7% of them are women. There are 12,286 young carers between the ages of 15 and 24 years and there is evidence to show that there are a significant number of children younger than 15 years of age who are also informal carers (Department of Health and Children 2010). The 2011 census included a question about young carers that will provide an accurate figure of the numbers of children who are caring on a regular basis. The total number of informal carers is much greater than the number of paid carers.

WHY CARE?

Care work is very satisfying, often for both parties. Most people who work in a care setting report feelings of satisfaction from working with vulnerable people. Personal needs such as feeling valued, raised self-esteem and fulfilling one's potential can be met by working as a carer. Assisting another person to live a more independent and autonomous existence, which will help that person to lead a more comfortable, independent and fulfilling life, is very rewarding.

> **Task**
>
> Make a list of your skills and qualities and write out the reasons why you want to be a health care worker.

ROLES

In everyday life, we all have different roles. Sometimes our roles change two or three times in a day – or even in an hour! As children we have no control over our roles within our families; as sons/daughters/grandchildren we accept the roles that we have and work within them, but as we grow older we make conscious decisions to undertake specific roles, such as applying for a job or becoming a parent. However, there are still times when we find ourselves in a role due to circumstances outside of our control, perhaps due to accident, illness or infirmity. This is when all options for care need to be considered and decisions made. There will be times when relationships will be supportive or dependent – for example, parents usually support their children – but at different stages, either through illness, disability or old age, the roles will be reversed and children will become supportive of their parents. A child with a disability may need a lifetime of care, so parents may look to their families initially for support but also to the wider community of health services and voluntary organisations.

For example, take a mother of a child with a disability. She may have other children with different needs or other roles to accommodate – how can she juggle all these roles? No matter what other roles she assumes, how can she maintain her own integrity?

Figure 7.1: Roles

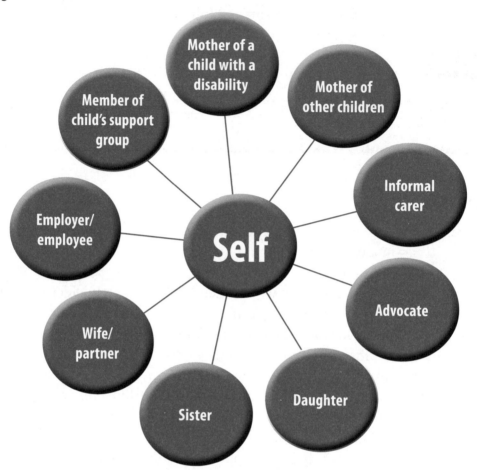

The same principle applies to CCAs – how can you retain your personal integrity when taking on the role of CCA? You have to accept that there are professional boundaries to be maintained and understanding appropriate communication regarding the client's gender, age and culture is also important, but there is no need to try to deny yourself when working in care practice. For example, if you are naturally quiet, there is no need to force yourself to be an extrovert, or if you are naturally an extrovert, there is no need to constantly bite your tongue.

Task

Take a few minutes to identify and write down your own roles in life. Consider how you behave similarly and differently within each role.

Just as we all have different roles in life, there are also different roles within the social model of health for the health care worker. What is significant for all of these roles is the close proximity that CCAs have in working with individuals and their families. You will need to be prepared to work on your own initiative as well as being part of a team and it is especially important to be flexibile when working with different client groups because of the varying needs of individuals and groups. While you need to have a good insight into and understanding of the individual in receipt of care and their needs, it is also important to have good personal understanding and insight. People interested in or undertaking care work need to be conscious of the qualities, attitudes, skills and values they bring to their care practice. Some qualities of a CCA might include being kind, caring, compassionate, understanding, altruistic and communicative as well as having a sense of humour. A CCA should be able to identify their own strengths and weaknesses and understand the impact they have on their practice and on the relationships with the people they come into contact with. It is important to work to stronger points and develop new or weaker ones.

COMMUNICATION

Good communication skills are essential for a CCA, including verbal, non-verbal and written communication. (See Chapter 6 for more detail on communcation.) Active listening is also integral to effective communication. The Greek philosopher Epictetus (55–135 AD) said, 'We have two ears and one mouth so that we can listen twice as much as we speak.'

PERSON-CENTRED CARE

Carl Rogers identified empathy, congruence and unconditional positive regard as three essential qualities for person-centred care. Empathy means the ability to understand someone else's feelings as if they were one's own. CCAs often have good insight and understanding into their client's situation, and this can be developed through experience, careful listening, consideration and respect for the client.

Congruence means similar or corresponding. For CCAs, this is the ability to work in line with what is usually espoused within legislation and national and organisational policy in order to assist and support clients in achieving their potential. It might be helpful to keep in mind the maxim 'treat others as you would like to be treated yourself'. It is understandable that CCAs can become tired and frustrated in their work, but it is not acceptable that the repercussions of this tiredness and frustration are perpetrated on people in their care. For example, if the organisational mission statement includes treating all people equally with dignity and respect and helping them to achieve their potential, that means always – not just on condition that the staff are not tired or frustrated.

Unconditional positive regard means being non-judgemental in care practice and treating everybody equally with high regard, no matter what their disposition, values or beliefs are. This can be quite difficult to uphold at times, but as a CCA you need to examine your own attitudes, values and beliefs. Because you will be caring for people with and from diverse cultures, traditions and beliefs, it is important to know where your own opinions and prejudices lie, not only to make any changes within yourself that may be necessary, but also to appreciate other people and situations and deliver respectful care.

Task

1. Where do your attitudes and beliefs come from? Are they from personal experience or popular beliefs that lead to negative stereotyping?
2. Have you ever said something like 'I don't want to sound racist/sexist/ageist, BUT...' and then continued to make a comment that *is* racist/sexist/ageist? Where is the line between a legitimate observation and a negative stereotypical comment?

ADVOCACY

One of the CCA's roles is to act as an advocate on behalf of the client. This is a difficult role, but it is integral to every health care profession. We choose to work with vulnerable people and therefore we must accept all aspects of the role. The individuals and their families face many dilemmas and they often discuss those issues with the CCA, who they know best. It is often said that the Irish are no good at complaining – we take what is given because we don't want to upset anyone or cause a row. Some people are assertive enough to advocate for themselves and others, some will not advocate on their own behalf but will have no problem advocating for another, more vulnerable person, while others will never advocate for fear of causing trouble. Knowing that advocacy is integral to caring means that CCAs who are more passive need to develop their assertiveness skills in order to advocate for the people in their care.

ISSUES FOR CARE WORKERS

A common theme running through this book is the necessity for carers to have a good knowledge and understanding of themselves, the people they are caring for and the theories or models of care that they employ in order to meet the needs of the individual. Two tools associated with personal and professional development are reflexivity and supervision, and formal processes in relation to them have long been integral elements in the fields of psychology, counselling and social work practice.

Kelleher and O'Donovan (2006: 20) identify a number of relevant issues for social care workers, as follows:

> *While you do not have any extra rights as a (social care) worker, you do have some extra needs; these include the need for training, supervision and support from co-workers and your supervisor.*

The combination of a number of events and developments in the field of social care, such as the many reports into abuse of vulnerable people, the professionalisation of social care (Health and Social Care Professional's Act 2005) and the work of HIQA, has resulted in changes being made.

Carers are now expected to be confident and competent in their care practice, but this cannot happen in a vacuum. In order to address the needs identified by Kelleher and O'Donovan (2006), and with the benefits associated with reflective practice and supervision well researched and acknowledged, CORU has included them across all health and social care professionals' education and training programmes, including those for social care workers. In this section, consideration is given to these practices.

There are links in this chapter with Chapter 1 on care provision and practice, so it is a good idea to review it, particularly the sections about the care worker and Erikson's stages of development, where you will notice that during adolescence and young adulthood, there is a focus firstly on self-development and then on interpersonal development, i.e. creating and maintaining relationships with others. These stages are hard work and sometimes difficult to negotiate, but when caring for vulnerable people, high levels of insight and awareness are important and a carer will need extra support and encouragement in their personal and professional development.

There are two useful adages to bear in mind here: 'we learn from our mistakes' and 'hindsight is 20/20'. However, for a variety of reasons, some people do not learn from their mistakes and they may continuously make poor decisions or they may not have learned because a situation was not explored adequately. Experiential learning, reflexivity and supervision are all elements of support.

REFLECTIVE PRACTICE

The study and ethos of adult education and lifelong learning have developed rapidly since the 1970s and there are now lifelong learning policies and strategies in place both internationally and locally. Many people have carried out research and developed theories about adult education, and all seem to agree on some key principles:

- People learn in a variety of different ways.
- Students should be supported in identifying their strongest method of learning, utilising their strengths and developing their weaknesses.
- Experiences and emotions play an important role in learning and need to be included in the learning process.
- Experiences without reflection do not necessarily create new learning.
- A problem-solving approach to learning helps students to connect actively with the process.
- Independence and autonomy in learning encourage students to transfer learning to practice.

These ideas are particularly relevant for carers because of their frontline work with vulnerable people, so it is important to understand and activate the process of reflective practice. There is a danger, as Brookfield (1995) points out, that:

The quantity or length of experience is not necessarily connected to its richness or intensity, for example, in an adult education career spanning thirty years the same, one year's experience can, in effect, be repeated thirty times.

This sentiment can be applied to a carer's career when the same daily tasks are performed without consideration for the external environment, for example a change in the mood, health and well-being of the individual receiving care, or even a change in the weather or weekends and bank holidays.

Reflection is something that many of us do automatically and informally, either while carrying out a task, during an encounter with somebody or after an event. Quite often, during an event or task we decide that the process is not going too well and immediately change direction or method (this is known as reflection-in-practice), whereas at other times, upon considering an earlier experience we might make a decision to act differently the next time we are in that sort of situation (this is known as reflection-on-practice). Learning and development occur in this context and this can be enhanced if there is a 'significant other' around, for example a parent, partner or teacher, to guide and lead through discussion and by example.

Another educational theorist, David Kolb (1984), suggested that 'learning is the process whereby knowledge is created through the transformation of experience'. He developed a model of experiential learning to demonstrate this process.

Figure 7.2: Experiential learning

Concrete experience
Doing/having an experience

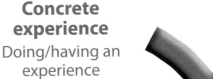

Reflective observation
Reviewing/reflecting on the experience

Abstract conceptualisation
Concluding/learning from experience

Active experimentation
Planning/trying out what you have learned

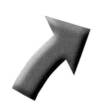

Source: Kolb (1984).

143

The experiential learning framework is usually illustrated in a cyclical or spiral style to demonstrate that reflexivity is continuous or ongoing and starts with identifying an experience, thinking about it, learning from it and planning and implementing new learning. Within each element there are a number of tasks that the practitioner should complete.

* **Concrete experience** – the feeling stage: This involves clearly describing the experience, including the actors and conversations involved in it, as well as being sensitive to your own and other people's feelings – do you know how the other people felt? How do you know?

* **Reflective observation** – the watching stage: Observing from a different perspective before passing judgement (for example, asking yourself how you would feel if you were receiving that type of care) involves reviewing or revisiting the experience and reflecting on it by questioning the outcomes of the event. What were the positive and negative aspects? Why did it conclude in the way it did?

* **Abstract conceptualisation** – the thinking stage: This involves logical analysis to gain an intellectual understanding of the situation. What information/knowledge did you have/need? Is there another way to do this? What are possible outcomes of other options? It involves learning from the experience.

* **Active experimentation** – the doing stage: This involves planning and implementing a new approach or method. This stage is the riskiest one, as it involves influencing people and events through action.

After reading this section and considering the different elements of reflexivity, the best way to engage with reflexivity is to consciously do it.

> **Task**
>
> 1. Identify a learning experience and reflect on it. For example, it could be learning to drive/cycle/knit or it could be related to care practice, e.g. learning to feed an adult, changing an occupied bed or communicating with a non-verbal person. Write down your considerations for each stage.
>
> 2. Identify a difficult past experience, professional or personal. Following the four stages of Kolb's cycle of experiential learning, ask yourself if you think differently about it now than you did then. Write down the different feelings, ideas and behaviours that you had at the time. Then write down what you would do now in the same situation. Consider why your opinion is different/the same. Have you identified any prejudices that you may have held then or still hold now? What knowledge, skills or qualities have you developed since then, if any?

MENTORING

While undertaking the reflective tasks, you may have noticed that your mind wandered off on a number of tangents or that you are not quite sure of the efficacy of the process. However, another point to consider is the fact that we often stay within our comfort zones and defend our actions and omissions (usually time and financial constraints) rather than ask ourselves the difficult questions and consider the situation from the other's perspective (for example, how it would be to be a recipient of your care practice). Furthermore, some situations are so difficult and complex that given the bounds of confidentiality in care practice being so important, burdens are placed on carers that are difficult to shoulder. Burnout occurs as a result of persistently high levels of responsibilities and stress. The individual feels powerless in their work, problems are unsolvable and the ability to care has diminished or even gone. Burnout amongst health care workers is high, with low staffing levels, lack of autonomy and independence in work and lack of formal supervision being cited as some of the reasons for this. Some research shows that levels of burnout are higher amongst frontline staff than amongst staff who are slightly removed from the situation. Within well-established fields of health care, such as psychotherapy and social work, supervision is routinely practised, whereas in social care it is a fairly recent addition. This is why recognition is now being given to the formal supervisory process in care practice.

The very term 'supervision' often has negative connotations. People generally relate it to a manager checking the standard of their practice to make sure that they are fulfilling all aspects of their employment contract. There may also be a link with appraisals where levels of efficiency are evaluated. There are different names that further complicate matters – clinical supervision, professional supervision, coaching and mentoring – with no clear understanding of distinctions or overlaps in meanings. For the purpose of this chapter, the term 'mentoring' will be used, as it fits nicely with frontline caring.

Mentoring is understood to be undertaken within a professional relationship whereby an experienced practitioner will support a less experienced one to develop skills, knowledge and information in order to enhance personal and professional development. The experienced person is the mentor and the less experienced person is the mentee.

There are a number of ways to mentor: group, peer, individual, formal and informal. Informal mentoring occurs frequently, for example sitting with peers or friends and discussing work or family-related issues and difficulties over a cup of tea and sharing ideas on overcoming them. As many will know, it is a valuable experience – 'a problem shared is a problem halved'. As with other elements of training and education for carers, this is about putting structures in place to formalise the process so that carers can be supported in their practice through learning.

Initially, individual or group mentoring seems to be practical for carers, as it reduces anxieties around the process. On the one hand, while individual mentoring allows for confidentiality between the mentor and mentee, the mentee may feel a little pressurised by the intensity of it, whereas group mentoring may be less intensive. Individuals may not be as open within a group setting, so there is usually a decision made based on the mentor's availability – maybe a compromise would be to begin with group mentoring and move on to individual mentoring.

The philosophy of mentoring is based on mutual respect within an equal relationship through which both will learn. Clarifying the responsibilities of both the mentor and the mentee will help to reduce the tension around mentoring.

The mentor has a number of responsibilities, including:

- Ensuring that the mentee is well trained and prepared to mentor
- Sharing knowledge and experience, particularly as they may have useful information relating to organisation-specific practices
- Assisting in the identification and setting of goals that are SMART (specific, measured, achievable, realistic and time-bound)
- Supporting the mentee through difficult phases with encouragement and positive feedback
- Using a problem-solving approach and identifying resources and tools for overcoming a specific problem.

The mentee also has a number of responsibilities, including:

- Being a willing participant and holding a positive outlook in relation to the process, viewing it as an opportunity for personal and professional development and entering into it with openness
- Taking responsibility for personal learning and using initiative for the progression of learning
- Identifying short-term and long-term goals as well as strategies for achieving them
- Taking risks (as linked with Kolb's final stage of experiential learning) and implementing new learning in practice, planned with and supported by the mentor.

The process involved in mentoring relates to establishing the structure, setting an agenda and timetable and agreeing the framework and ground rules.

BENEFITS OF SUPERVISION

Many studies into the benefits of good supervision identify categories that the benefits fall into: the organisation, the multidisciplinary team, staff and the recipients of care. Effective communication, role/boundary clarity, improved confidence and self-esteem, personal support (i.e. the practice, learning and emotional needs of staff are acknowledged and addressed), an increase in evidence-based practice, improved understanding of power structures and higher involvement with the organisation all translates to lower staff turnover and makes recruitment and continuity of care easier. The end result, of course, is that carers achieve the aim of becoming confident and competent in their care practice and deliver a high standard of care – which is what the individual in receipt of care is entitled to.

BARRIERS TO SUPERVISION

Organisations will often cite time and money as barriers to training mentors and implementing supervision, but there are other reasons why mentoring is unsatisfactory when it is in place, including poor preparation of either the mentor/mentee or the process; lack of privacy and constant interruptions; lack of adequate recording of the process; confusion relating to management and mentoring, with a focus on management and appraisals rather than professional/personal development; and little attention to quality assurance.

Task

1. Who supported and guided you through your childhood and teenage years? In what way did it happen? Through discussion? Through example? Through your own experiences?
2. Consider the decisions you made and the responsibilities you had in your late teens and early twenties. What was the personal impact of them?

SUMMARY

In this chapter, a range of topics associated with care practice has been explored to highlight the connections between personal and professional development within care practice. These topics include the role of the CCA, how the qualities, skills, values, beliefs and attitudes of the CCA impact on individuals in receipt of care, experiential learning, reflective practice and mentoring.

This is the final chapter in the book, as care practice is the culmination of the Community and Health Services Award. It is hoped that by integrating the knowledge, skills and qualities that you have explored during the course, you will be confident and competent in your practice.

REFERENCES

Brookfield, S. (1995) 'Adult Learning: An Overview' in A. Tuinjman (ed.), *International Encyclopedia of Education*, Oxford: Pergamon Press.

Department of Health and Children (2010) *National Children's Strategy Research Series – Study of Young Carers in the Irish Population*, Dublin: Government Publications.

Kelleher, C. and O'Donovan, O. (2006) *Redefining Health and Wellbeing*, 2nd edition, Galway: Health Promotion Research Centre, National University of Ireland.

Kolb, D.A. (1984) *Experiential Learning: Experience as the Source of Learning and Development*, Englewood Cliffs, NJ: Prentice-Hall.

Index

A

A Vision for Change: Report of the Expert Group on Mental Health Policy, 102

Ability Awards, 91

abuse, 45–8, 141

acceptance, 120

access, 55–6, 58, 86–7, 89, 91

Access Officers, 90

accommodation, reasonable, 55, 90

accountability, 119

acquired brain injuries, 62–4

active listening, 121, 129–30, 139

adult education, 142

advocacy, 128, 140–1

affective disorders, 109

Age Action Ireland, 31, 33

ageing

  body appearance, 34

  factors in, 32–4

  healthy, 29, 30, 33

  mobility, 34–5

  as social construction, 30

  see also older people

Alzheimer's disease, 38, 41, 72, 74

Alzheimer's Society of Ireland, 31, 41

anti-discriminatory practice, 92–4

  see also discrimination, disabled people

anti-psychotic drugs, 113

anxiety, 101, 109

aphasia, 133

Asperger's syndrome, 76

assessment, 20, 25–6, 130–1

assistive technology, 67, 68, 95–7

asylum seekers, 21

asylums, 100, 101

attitudes

  discriminatory, 86, 88–9, 93

  needed for care work, 124–5

auras, 60

autism, 74–7, 88

Aware, 103

B

balance, 37

Bedlam, 100

bereavement, 49–50

Berglund, C. A., 44

biopsychosocial model, 106–7

bipolar disorder, 109

Black Report, 11, 12

blindness, 57, 66–7, 72, 133, 137

body language, 129

bones, 35

brain injuries, 62–4

Brookfield, S., 142

buccal midazolam, 60

burnout, 145

C

cardiovascular disease, 35, 38, 49, 72

care plans, 23, 25, 27, 38, 131–2

care work
  attitudes needed for, 124–5
  objectivity, 119
  versus personal care, 117–19
  person-centred care, 23, 40, 139–40
  power relations, 119, 127
  recipients of, 22–3
  reflective practice, 141
  relationships, 129
  rewards from, 136–7
  roles, 137–9
  types of, 138–9
  values and principles, 124–5
carers, 130, 136
Casey, Caroline, 91
cataracts, 37, 66, 74
Cavan County Council, 91
cerebral palsy, 61–2
challenging behaviour, 77–80
chronic obstructive pulmonary disease
    (COPD), 36, 49
client-centred therapy, 112–13
coeliac disease, 4, 72
colloquialisms, 133
communication
  active listening, 121, 129–31, 139
  in assessment, 130
  autism, 74, 75
  barriers to, 132–3
  challenging behaviour, 77–8
  dementia, 41–2
  older people, 44, 49, 125
  therapeutic, 3, 43, 117, 139
community care assistants
  attitudes required, 124–5
  key skills, 118, 120–1, 139
  roles, 136, 137–9
  training, 128
community development, 14–15
conditional love, 112

confidentiality, 24, 44, 121–4
congruence, 112, 129, 139–40
contracts, 130
COPD (chronic obstructive pulmonary
    disease), 36, 49
Corcoran, M., 40
culture, 20
cutbacks, 87
  see also recession

D
daily living, activities, 23
Dara Has the Craic, 91–2
data protection, 123–4
Data Protection Commissioner, 123
deafness, 37, 67–8, 133
death, 48–50
dementia
  communication, 41–2
  environmental factors, 40
  learning disabilities, 40–1
  palliative care, 49
  symptoms, 39, 40, 74
  types, 38–9
Dementia Services Information and
    Development Centre, 38
depression, 49, 50, 109, 110–11
detention centres, 8
development
  Erik Erikson's stages, 17–19, 26, 141–2
  pervasive developmental disorders,
    74–7
diabetes, 64–6
diagnosis, 27
*Diagnostic and Statistical Manual of Mental
    Disorders (DSM)*, 105
diazepam, 60
Dickson, D., 125
dieticians, 4
digestive system, 36

disabilities
  acquired brain injuries, 62–4
  definitions, 20, 53–4, 86
  discriminatory attitudes and barriers,
    86, 88–90, 92–4
  emotional/psychological, 57
  hearing, 57, 67–8, 133
  hidden, 64–6, 77
  integrated services, 55
  intellectual *see* intellectual disabilities
  in Ireland, 54, 85–6
  learning disabilities, 21–2, 40–1
  legislation, 55–6, 86
  physical, 21, 57–62
  prevalence, 55
  and social exclusion, 54, 85–7
  social model, 9, 22, 23, 54–5, 139
  speech, 57
  types, 21–2, 55–6, 86
  visual, 37, 57, 66–7, 72, 133
Disability Act 2005, 20, 55–6, 86, 87
Disability and Social Inclusion in Ireland,
  85–6
discrimination
  attitudes, 86, 88–9, 93
  disabled people, 55, 86, 88–90, 92–4
Down syndrome, 41, 69, 71–4
Downie, R. S., 13–14
Drug Payment Scheme, 31
drugs, anti-psychotic, 113
*DSM (Diagnostic and Statistical Manual of
  Mental Disorders)*, 105

E
Economic and Social Research Institute,
  11
education
  adult education, 142
  integrated, 55, 90
  special education, 55, 92

Egan, G., 129
elder abuse, 45–8
Emerson, E., 78
emotional abuse, 45, 46, 47
emotional disabilities, 57
emotional health, 10, 42–3, 50
empathy, 43, 112, 120, 121, 129, 139
Employment Equality Acts, 90
empowerment, 14, 27, 42, 89, 119, 127–8
Epictetus, 139
epilepsy, 58–61
equal opportunities, 91–4
  see also discrimination
Equal Status Act 2000, 90
Equality Authority, 91
Erikson, Erik, 17–19, 26, 141
Esterson, A., 104
ethnicity, 20
European Year of People with Disabilities,
  54
Ewles, L., 9–10, 42
Excellence through Accessibility Award,
  86–7
existential perspective, 111
experiential learning, 135, 142, 143–4,
  147
eye problems, 37, 57, 66–7, 72, 133

F
Fair Deal scheme, 31
falls, 35
families, 104
files, 122
financial abuse, 45, 47
fits, epileptic, 58–61
flexible working, 103
foster care, 8
Freire, Paulo, 127
functional psychoses, 108–9

G

general nurses (RGNs), 4
general practitioners (GPs), 4
Gitlin, L., 40
glaucoma, 37, 66, 72
Grow, 103
Gudykunst, W., 125

H

Hargie, O., 125
health
  care *see* health care
  definitions, 11, 12, 99–100
  determinants, 11
  dimensions, 9–19, 42
  holistic perspective, 11–12, 42, 111
  information, 8
    see also Health Information and
      Quality Authority (HIQA)
  medical model, 2, 9, 22
  mental health *see* mental health; mental
    illness
  physical, 9, 25–6
  promotion, 12–14, 34
  sexual, 9
  social health, 10
  social model, 2–3, 9, 22, 23
  spiritual health, 10, 26
  technology, 8
Health Act 2007, 31
Health and Social Care Council, 3
Health and Social Care Professional's Act
  2005, 3, 141
Health Boards, 6
health care
  history, 1–3
  holistic perspective, 11–12
  information *see* Health Information and
    Quality Authority (HIQA)
  legislation and policy, 5–6

organisations, 6–7
quality assurance, 7–8, 31 *see also*
    Health Information and Quality
    Authority (HIQA)
health care assistants, 4
  see also community care assistants
Health Information and Quality Authority
    (HIQA)
  dementia, 38
  equality in care, 92
  principles of social care, 23
  residential care, 127, 128
  responsibilities, 7–8, 31
Health Service Executive, 4, 30, 31
healthy ageing, 29, 30, 33
hearing disabilities, 57, 67–8, 133
heart disease/failure, 35, 38, 49, 72
helplessness, learned, 126–7
hidden disabilities, 64–6, 77
hierarchy of needs, 15–17, 26, 112
HIQA (Health Information and Quality
    Authority) *see* Health Information and
    Quality Authority (HIQA)
holistic perspective
  care work, 70
  health, 11–12, 42, 111
Home Care Packages, 31
Home for Good, 41
Howlin, Brendan, 6
humanistic perspective, 15, 111–14
hypothyroidism, 72, 74

I

ICD (International Classification of Mental
    and Behavioural Disorders), 105
impairments, 53–4
  see also disability
Inclusion Ireland, 22–3, 87
independence, 24, 50, 77
informal carers, 136

information
  accessible forms, 55, 87
  confidential, 122–4
  health, 8 *see also* Health Information
      and Quality Authority (HIQA)
insulin, 64
integration, 55, 90
intellectual disabilities
  autism, 74–7, 88
  care management, 70
  causes, 69
  challenging behaviour, 77–80
  Down syndrome, 71–4
  education and training, 87
  learning disabilities, 21–2, 40–1
  National Association for People with an
      Intellectual Disability, 22–3
  nature, 68–9
  prevalence, 57
International Classification of Mental and
    Behavioural Disorders (ICD), 105
International Telecommunication Union,
    95
interpersonal skills, 43, 44

J
joints, 35

K
Kanchi, 91
Katz, D., 125
Kelleher, C., 141
Kenny, Enda, 58
Kerr, D., 40–1
Kildare County Council, 91
Kolb, David, 143, 147

L
Laing, R., 104
Langer, E. J., 126–7

language, 88
learned helplessness, 126–7
learning disabilities, 21–2, 40–1
  see also intellectual disabilities
legislation
  data protection, 123
  disability, 54, 55–6, 86, 87, 89, 90
  health, 3, 5–6, 102, 141
lifelong learning, 142
listening, active, 121, 129–30, 139
London 2012 Paralympics, 58, 91
lung diseases, 35–6

M
manic depression, 109
Maslow, Abraham, 15–17, 26, 111,
    112
Medical Card, 31
medical model, 2, 9, 22
memory, 38, 39, 42, 63, 108, 111
mental health
  causes, 106–7
  definition, 10, 99–100, 105–6
  humanistic perspective, 111–12
  promotion, 103–4
  see also mental illness
Mental Health Act 2001, 102
Mental Health Commission, 102
mental illness
  anxiety, 101, 109
  attitudes to, 88
  causes, 104–5
  depression, 49, 50, 109, 110–11
  diagnosis, 105–6
  history of care, 100–1
  humanistic perspective, 111–14
  legislation and policy, 102
  neurosis, 110–11
  personality disorders, 110
  prevalence, 57, 64

prevention *see* mental health, promotion
psychosis, 88, 107–9, 113
psychosocial interventions, 113–14
services, 102–3
types, 22
see also mental health
mentoring, 145–8
mobility, 34–5, 42, 56
Monastery of St Mary of Bethlehem in London, 100
Morrissey, J., 113
motivation, 126–7
multidisciplinary teams, 2–4, 31–2
multiple schlerosis, 37

N
National Association for People with an Intellectual Disability, 22–3
National Disability Strategy, 55, 86
National Disability Survey 2006, 56–7
National Office for Suicide Prevention, 101–2
Naughton, C., 45
neglect, 45, 47
neurological disorders, 37
neurosis, 110–11
nurses, 4
Nursing Homes Support Scheme, 31
nursing process, 24–7

O
obesity, 4, 35, 72, 74
objectivity, in care work, 119
occupational therapists, 4
O'Donovan, O., 141
older people
communication with, 44, 49, 125
death and dying, 48–50
definition, 21, 29–30

emotional development, 42–3, 50
empowerment, 127
good practice in care, 43
mobility, 42
residential care, 8
safeguarding, 45–8
services, 30–2
stereotyping, 125
operant conditioning, 78
organic psychoses, 108
O'Riordan, Joanne, 58, 80, 91, 95–7
osteoarthritis, 35
osteoporosis, 35
Ottawa Charter, 12–13

P
pain, 41, 57
palliative care, 48–9
Paralympics, London 2012, 58, 91
pensions, 31
permission, 24
personality disorders, 110
person-centred care, 23, 40, 139–40
pervasive developmental disorders, 74–7
phenomenological perspective, 111
phobias, 109
physical abuse, 45
physical disabilities, 21, 57–62
physical health, 9, 25–6
physiotherapists, 4
Pinel, Philippe, 101
policy, health, 5–6
positive behaviour support, 79–80
positive reinforcement, 78–9
poverty, 86
power relations, in care work, 119, 127
prejudices, 140
see also attitudes, discriminatory
pre-school services, 8

primary care teams, 31–2
privacy, 24, 44, 121
private sector organisations, 7, 103
Programme for National Recovery, 87
Programme for Prosperity and Fairness
    Agreement, 86–7
psychological abuse, 45, 46, 47
psychological disabilities, 57
psychosis, 107–9, 113
psychosocial interventions, 113–14
public health nurses, 4

Q
quality assurance, 7–8, 31
    see also Health Information and Quality
        Authority (HIQA)

R
Reach Out – National Strategy for Action on
    Suicide Prevention, 102
reasonable accommodation, 55, 90
recession, 104
    see also cutbacks
records, 131
reflective practice, 141, 142–4
refugees, 21
registered nurse intellectual disability
    (RNID), 4
registered nurses, 4
registered psychiatric nurses (RPN), 4
relationships, in care work, 129
reliability, 121
religious beliefs, 10
residential care
    abuse, 45
    contracts, 130
    empowering residents, 126–7
    equality in care, 92
    health promotion, 34
    inspection, 8, 31

respect, 121
respiratory illnesses, 35–6, 49, 57
retirement, 33, 34
RNID (registered nurse intellectual
    disability), 4
Rodin, J., 126–7
Rogers, Carl, 15, 111, 112, 129, 139
roles, in care work, 137–9
RPN (registered psychiatric nurses), 4

S
Saltman, D., 44
schizophrenia, 88, 107, 108–9, 113
Schriven, A., 42
segregation, 54
seizures, epileptic, 58–61
self-actualisation, 17, 112
self-esteem, 17
self-harm, 78, 101–2
sensory disabilities, 66–8
sexual abuse, 45, 46
sexual behaviour, 72–3, 78
sexual health, 9
Shaping a Healthier Future, 6, 7
Sheridan, A., 100–1
Shine, 103
sight problems, 37, 57, 66–7, 72,
    133
Simnett, I., 9–10, 42
Skinner, B. F., 78
sleep patterns, 42
social care, principles, 23
social exclusion, 54, 85–7
social health, 10
social model, 9, 22, 23, 54–5, 139
Social Service Inspectorate, 8
social workers, 4
societal health, 10
special education, 55, 90
speech disabilities, 57

spiritual groups, 50
spiritual health, 10, 26
Spring, B., 107
standards, health care, 8
status epilepticus, 59–60
statutory organisations, 6, 103
stereotyping, 73, 77, 85, 88–9, 93, 125
stigma, 55, 60–1, 89, 100, 101, 103
Stotland, E., 125
stress vulnerability model, 107
students, 122
suicide, 101–2
supervision, 141, 145–8

T
Tannahill, A. and C., 13–14
tardive dyskinesia, 113
tetrogens, 69
therapeutic communication, 3, 43, 117, 139
therapy, client-centred, 112–13
Ting-Toomey, S., 125
total amelia syndrome, 91, 95
training, community care assistants, 128
Travellers, 20
triad of impairments, autism, 75
Tyas, S. L., 33

U
unconditional positive regard, 112, 129, 139, 140
unemployment, 86

V
values and principles, care work, 124–5
Vision for Change, 22
visual disabilities, 37, 57, 66–7, 72, 133
voluntary organisations, 6–7, 103

W
Wilkinson, H., 41
work placements, 122, 135
World Health Organization (WHO)
   definition of disability, 53–4
   definition of health, 11, 99–100
   health promotion, 12
   older people, 29

Y
young people, 5, 19, 101, 119

Z
Zaretsky, E., 133
Zubin, J., 107